SURVIVING
MALE
MENOPAUSE

A Guide for Women and Men

Jed Diamond

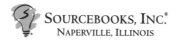

SOURCEBOOKS, INC.®
NAPERVILLE, ILLINOIS

This publication is designed to provide accurate and authoritative information in regard to the subject matter covered. It is sold with the understanding that the publisher is not engaged in rendering legal, accounting, or other professional service. If legal advice or other expert assistance is required, the services of a competent professional person should be sought.—*From a Declaration of Principles Jointly Adopted by a Committee of the American Bar Association and a Committee of Publishers and Associations*

Published by Sourcebooks, Inc.
P.O. Box 4410, Naperville, Illinois 60567-4410
(630) 961-3900
FAX: (630) 961-2168

Library of Congress Cataloging-in-Publication Data
Diamond, Jed, 1943–
    Surviving male menopause: a guide for women and men / Jed
    Diamond. p. cm.
    Includes bibliographical references and index.
    ISBN 1-57071-433-9 (alk. paper)
    1. Climateric, Male—Popular works. 2. Middle aged men—Health and
    hygiene—Popular works. I. Title

RC884.D525 2000
616.6'93—dc21   00-041979

Printed and bound in the United States of America
VHG 10 9 8 7 6 5 4 3 2 1

Acknowledgments

No book gets written without a tremendous amount of help and support. This is my opportunity to thank some of the key people who made it possible for you to hold the book you now have in your hands.

Carlin: Wife, lover, friend, colleague. She stayed and supported me during one of the most difficult times of my life. If you wonder whether male menopause is real, you need only ask Carlin. She knew I was going through "the change" long before I was aware of it. She helped me see that the anger and depression that are so much a part of this stage of life for many men need to be dealt with honestly and directly.

Nancy Ellis: My agent, friend, confidant, and supporter. She believes in my work during the good times and the dark times, and never fails to express her care and spirit of adventure.

Sourcebooks: Once again, the people at Sourcebooks have done a masterful job in getting the book ready for the readers, promoting it so that it reaches the right audience, and giving me the support to present these ideas to all those who are ready to hear them.

The women and men who are going through this stage of life and have the courage to face the change together: Thank you from the bottom of my heart for the calls, letters, emails, and support. I've been contacted by women and men from all over the world. Your response makes me know that this work is worthwhile and that men and women can look forward to menopause as the transition to the most passionate, powerful, and purposeful time of life we have yet experienced.

Thank you all.

Contents

Introduction

When I first started working on *Male Menopause* over ten years ago, very few people were aware that men, like women, experience hormonal and physiological changes that affect all aspects of their lives. I found that male menopause was a multi-dimensional life transition and could only be treated effectively by focusing on the hormonal, physical, psychological, interpersonal, social, spiritual, and sexual changes that occur in all men's lives.

In the past, many told us that male menopause didn't exist. Some saw it as a cheap attempt to steal attention or even funds from women dealing with their midlife problems. Others saw it as a way for women to "feminize" men and saddle them with the same midlife problems that were plaguing women. Some saw it as an attempt by the medical and pharmaceutical establishments to create a new disease that would allow them to sell new drugs and make more profits. Others felt it was a way for men to justify leaving their aging wives and the responsibilities of midlife to run off with a young beauty and buy all the toys they never had as young men.

I don't think this is why there is such an interest in male menopause as we enter the twenty-first century. The baby boomers, who are now moving into the menopause years, are a health-oriented generation. Men, as well as women, want to share in the benefits of living long, healthy, and satisfying lives. Male menopause is the transition period that prepares us for life in the second half. How well we move through this period will determine what our lives will be like when we are fifty, sixty, seventy, eighty, ninety, and one hundred years old.

In writing *Male Menopause*, I drew on the latest information from my own clinical experience over the last thirty-five years, as well as from worldwide studies on sexuality, longevity, and vitality medicine. I introduced you to a new medication, sildenafil citrate (marketed as Viagra). It was hoped that this new drug would help the hundreds of millions of men throughout the world who were suffering from erectile dysfunction (ED).

Although Viagra became an instant success, it didn't solve all the problems that men were experiencing. While it did a good job in helping men restore lost erections, it didn't help men with their loss of sexual desire, increased fatigue, added depression and anger, and loss of muscle strength and bone mass.

For many years, researchers have wondered whether men, like women, would benefit from hormone replacement therapy. At the First World Congress on the Aging Male held in 1998, Bruno Lunenfeld, M.D., president of the International Society for the Study of the Aging Male, said, "Evidence is available that such interventions reduce cardiovascular disease and osteoporosis and may delay the onset of Alzheimer's disease in women. There is an urgent need to obtain such information in men."

Two years later, at the Second World Congress, research is mounting that testosterone replacement therapy may be helpful in preventing many of the problems associated with male menopause. One of the world experts on testosterone and male menopause is Dr. John E. Morley, chairman of the Department of Geriatric Medicine at St. Louis University School of Medicine. "Low testosterone with aging is responsible for a decline in cognition, strength, bone density, and sexual drive," says Dr. Morley. He notes that testosterone replacement is helpful in treating these symptoms. He also says that testosterone replacement may have positive effects on cardiovascular disease and osteoporosis in older males.

Dr. Morley developed a simple questionnaire which can be used as a screening tool for testosterone deficiency.

1. Do you have a decrease in libido (sex drive)?
2. Do you have a lack of energy?
3. Do you have a decrease in strength and/or endurance?
4. Have you lost height?
5. Have you noticed a decreased "enjoyment of life"?
6. Are you sad and/or grumpy?
7. Are your erections less strong?
8. Have you noticed a recent deterioration in your ability to play sports?
9. Are you falling asleep after dinner?
10. Has there been a recent deterioration in your work performance?

Answering yes to these questions does not mean you are simply getting old and must accept these changes.

If you answer yes to questions 1 or 7 and/or yes to any three other questions, there is evidence that you are suffering from testosterone deficiency and should have your bio-available testosterone levels checked.

If it is determined that testosterone replacement therapy should be part of the total program for treating male menopause, there are a number of ways testosterone can be administered. It can be given by injection usually every two to three weeks. Testosterone pellets can be implanted and last for three to four months. There are also testosterone patches—Testoderm, which is placed directly on the scrotum, and Androderm, which is placed on other parts of the body.

AndroGel is a new preparation that was released in the summer of 2000. It is a gel that can be rubbed directly into the skin and restores testosterone for men who are deficient.

Andriol is an oral preparation that is available in Europe and Canada and is expected to be offered in the U.S. in a few years.

Hormone replacement for men has been neglected in the U.S. However, with more research showing the importance of hormones, particularly testosterone, for helping men move through male menopause, there will be increasing interest. "His and her" hormone replacement therapy may become as common as "love and marriage." Though hormonal changes are not the only aspects of male menopause that need to be addressed, they are critical and are often neglected.

After writing *Male Menopause*, I received thousands of letters from women with a similar message: "You've described my husband perfectly. You must have written that book just for us. But I still don't understand him. Why is he so withdrawn and angry? Why has he turned off to me? What is he looking for? Why would he be willing to run off with a younger woman and destroy our family in a frantic search for what...his lost youth, his flagging manhood, what?"

I wrote *Surviving Male Menopause* to answer the many questions women and men have about what is going on with men during this crucial midlife period. More importantly, I want you to know what you can do to maintain your own peace of mind and protect your relationship. You can think of this book as a companion volume to *Male Menopause*.

In *Male Menopause*, you learned about the scientific basis for male menopause and the hormonal, psychological, social, and sexual changes that accompany this period in a man's life. In *Surviving Male Menopause*, you will be taken behind the scenes to experience what men and women are really going through. You will learn about the important questions such as how male menopause differs from the midlife crisis and aging, why men are so angry and depressed at this time of life, why men want to leave their wives or have affairs, the best methods for treating erectile dysfunction, and how to get through male menopause in the most loving way possible.

In *Surviving Male Menopause*, you will learn the essence of what it means to be a man and about the stages of manhood. You will learn why menopausal men act so much like adolescent boys and why it is so difficult for them to admit that they are going through a change of life every bit as important as what women experience.

You will learn what you can do to help them move through male menopause and how to take care of yourself along the way. You will understand the meaning of male menopause and how it can prepare a man to enter the most powerful, productive, and passionate time of his life. Finally, you will find out what it takes to make this journey together and to develop a relationship that can grow and change over time. You will find that the struggles are worthwhile and that the best is yet to come.

Your comments and questions are appreciated. I will try and answer each one. You can get more information on this work, other books and tapes, conferences and training events, and upcoming programs by contacting me on my website: www.MenAlive.com, or write to:

Jed Diamond
34133 Shimmins Ridge Rd.
Willits, CA 95490
Email: Jed@MenAlive.com

Chapter 1

Behind the Scenes

An Inside and Personal
Look at Male Menopause

When I began the research for my first book, *Male Menopause*, I was skeptical about the concept itself. I had been a therapist for more than thirty years and had worked with thousands of midlife men and women. Most of the women who were approaching menopause experienced marked changes that were related to physiological and hormonal shifts in body chemistry.

It was clear to me that something was also going on with the men, but I assumed that men's changes were more psychological than physical. I had heard a number of men and women talk about "male menopause," but wondered if they were just complaining about the difficulties of being a man or trying to justify their irresponsible midlife behavior. In a society where more and more people see themselves as victims, "my hormones made me do it," is not a surprising excuse.

As a therapist, I have little tolerance for men (or women) who bemoan their lives or who blame bad behavior on someone or something other than themselves. However, after completing ten years of research, I concluded that midlife men have significant hormonal and physiological changes as they move from the first half of life to the second.

The term "male menopause" itself, of course, is an oxymoron. Men don't have a menstrual cycle and so don't "stop" having one. But, after working with men for the last thirty-five years, I believe there is a deeper truth about the hormonal and physiological changes that occur for men at midlife that if not understood can be devastating to a man and his family.

It's time we broke the silence and began talking about the fact that men, too, go through a "change of life," because until we do, too many men will be struck down by disease, too many marriages will break up just when the couple has time to enjoy them the most, and too many men will die before their time.

Though there are still those who find the idea of "male menopause" about as ludicrous as "male menstrual cramps," more and more people are coming to recognize the reality of this universal male life passage. Although I had been working with midlife men for some time and had thought about the idea of male menopause, a magazine article helped direct my interest.

While perusing my local bookstore one day, I was drawn to a copy of *Vanity Fair* magazine. Well, to be absolutely honest, I was drawn to the cover photo of Sharon Stone, nude to the waist, with her hands cupping her breasts. Sharon was staring seductively into the eyes of the reader, with two inch letters blazoned across her bare midriff proclaiming, "Wild Thing!" Being a midlife man and fancying myself a bit of a wild man myself, I was sure there was something important that Sharon had to tell me.

However, I never read the article to find out, for just to the left of Sharon's blond hair, right below the April 1993 date line, were the words that grabbed me by the throat (actually a bit farther south than my throat)—"*Male Menopause: The Unspeakable Passage* by Gail Sheehy." Those words spoke in a quiet, but insistent voice. Inside I devoured the article "Is There a Male Menopause?" Sheehy said, "If menopause is the silent passage, 'male menopause' is the unspeakable passage. It is fraught with secrecy, shame, and denial."

I knew I had to continue my research on the changes that midlife men experience. I needed to find answers for myself and for the thousands of men and women who struggle to make sense of their lives at midlife.

This book, along with its companion *Male Menopause*, will give you the information you need to understand this vital period in a man's life. Since this is such a personal journey, I'd like to tell you a little bit more about myself and how male menopause burst on the national scene.

Dear Abby and Male Menopause

I'm a fifty-six-year-old, married man. My wife, Carlin, and I have been together more than twenty years and have raised our youngest two children together. We have five children in all and seven wonderful grandchildren. We have both been through each others' "change of life" and have learned some things along the way that we hope will be helpful to others. As a psychotherapist who has specialized in working with thousands of men and women over the last thirty-five years, I have had ample opportunity to learn about male menopause and how it differs from what women go through. I also have been able to find the common threads of experience that unite us all as we make the transition from what I call the Mountain of First Adulthood to the Mountain of Second Adulthood.

When I wrote *Male Menopause*, few people really understood what it was and how it affected men, women, and families. Since the book came out, I have received hundreds of letters from people all over the world attesting to the reality of male menopause in their lives. But it wasn't until a chance encounter with Abigail Van Buren, "Dear Abby," that the flow of response turned into a real flood.

I don't usually read Dear Abby, but this letter caught my eye one day.

Dear Abby:

I am a fifty-year-old man who has been married for twenty-two years. My wife and I have two wonderful teen-aged children.

About six months ago, my wife's niece (I'll call her Rene), whom I had never met, came from another country to live with us so she could go to college in the United States. She is in her early twenties.

For the first few months, everything was fine. Now I find myself thinking about Rene all the time. I think I'm in love with her. I travel quite a bit because of my job and every time I come home, it's torture. I have to act as if nothing is going on in my mind. No one knows the way I feel.

If I tell my wife, she'll be crushed and it will be the end of our marriage. If I tell Rene—who has done nothing wrong and loves my wife like a mother—she may want to return to her country without finishing her studies.

I have always tried to do the right thing. I never thought at this age I'd be feeling this way. I don't want to ruin anyone's life, including my own. What should I do?

Desperate in Delaware

Abby's response was clear and direct.

Dear Desperate:

Although it's common for older men to fantasize about younger women, the consequences of your fantasy could irreparably damage at least five lives. Talking this out with someone you trust would be helpful. I recommend a professional therapist, who can help you assess the consequences of acting out this fantasy.

I was pleasantly surprised that my response ran under a headline for her column which appeared in newspapers all over the country:

SYMPTOMS OF MALE MENOPAUSE ARE REAL

Dear Abby,

Thank you for the sensitive response to Desperate in Delaware, a fifty-year-old man with an obsessive attraction to a younger woman.

I have been a psychotherapist for thirty years and have seen too many men destroy their own lives and the lives of those they love because they didn't understand the inevitable changes that go on in a man's body, mind, and spirit at midlife.

I've found that my understanding of these issues has been greatly expanded since recognizing that men go through a form of "male menopause," generally between the ages of forty and fifty-five. Marc Blackman, M.D., chief of endocrinology and metabolism at Johns Hopkins Bayview Medical Center says, "The male menopause is a real phenomenon and it does similar things to men as menopause does to women, although less commonly and to a lesser extent."

I believe thousands of families could be saved from splitting apart if men and women learned about the newest research findings on this crucial time of life.

• More than twenty-five million men in the U.S. are now going through male menopause.

• Fifty-two percent of men between forty and seventy suffer from some degree of erectile dysfunction.

• Men, like women, experience complex hormonal rhythms that affect their mood, their physical well-being, and their sexuality.

• Emotional symptoms include irritability, worry, indecisiveness, and depression.

• Physical symptoms include fatigue, weight gain, short-term memory loss, and sleep disturbances.

• Sexual symptoms include reduced libido, fear of sexual failure, and increased desire to "prove" he can still perform by seeking a younger partner.

• All problems are treatable and help is available.

Jed Diamond

Abby's response was also clear and direct:

Dear Jed: Over the years, the idea that men experience a midlife change has been joked about. I'm sure many people will be relieved, and others will be surprised, to learn that male menopause is a fact and it is treatable.

Life and the Journey on the Two Mountains

I've always liked the idea of climbing mountains, though I never liked the idea that only those who make it to the top are worthy of praise or can claim success for themselves. How about just enjoying the journey? Going up and coming down and watching animals along the way and resting beside a clear mountain stream and being tired and exhilarated and stopping for a lunch that never tasted so good and finally reaching your destination or maybe ending up somewhere else than where you thought you'd be. Life is full of surprises.

But if life is like a mountain, the journey up and down was quite fast for most of human history. As late as 1910, the average life expectancy at birth in the United States was fifty years, slightly lower for males, a bit higher for females. Now, more and more people are living healthy and productive lives into our sixties, seventies, eighties, and beyond. "Virtually everyone has died too soon," says Walter M. Bortz II, M.D., author of *Dare to Be 100*. "Ours is the first generation in history to know what a whole human life can look like." It's clear that there is an exciting new life ahead of us, a second mountain to explore. But first we need to overcome our fear of going down into the valley between the two mountains.

Just Knowing What Is Happening Is a Major Relief

I have been struggling with all facets of my life lately. Everything from not enjoying the things I have always enjoyed, to losing my latest girlfriend over unknown reasons of which erectile dysfunction at some level was a factor. I have had problems with just everyday living, confusion, and lack of direction in my life. I happened across your book a couple days ago. Wow! What an enlightenment! Just knowing what is happening is a major relief and reduction in a very high level of anxiety. What do I do now?

Rob

Points of understanding:

• Often, male menopause begins slowly at first, speeds up, then all of a sudden it feels like the roof is caving in and everything is happening at once. It is very frightening to men and women when they are not expecting it.

• If not dealt with directly, it can cause a great deal of pain and create enough stress in a relationship to cause it to fall apart.

• The first step in dealing with it is to know it exists and what is happening hormonally, physically, emotionally, sexually, and spiritually.

• The next steps involve recognition that this is a normal, though painful, life transition and with guidance everyone can get through it and move on to the joys of second adulthood.

Since most of us have been taught that there is only one mountain in life, when we start coming down the backside we are sure we are getting close to death. It is no wonder that we fear the menopause passage like the plague. We avoid looking at it, hoping that if we turn our heads to the past we can stay forever young. As a result, many of us fail to understand this important transition period in our lives and fail to learn the lessons that would allow us to move up the second mountain of life with exuberance and passion. Though at fifty we may be an elder on the first mountain, we are just being born to the second. Exploring male menopause can give us the clues we need to construct a treasure map for the journey ahead.

I began to see the changes in myself as well as in friends and men I counseled, though at first the changes scared me and I tried to keep them concealed from everyone, including myself.

As I listened to friends and clients, men in their forties and fifties, I heard similar concerns about physical, emotional, and sexual changes. Many, like me, had been afraid to look closely at this time of life, but when given the opportunity to break the silence and talk with other men, they were eager.

"I have to wear bifocals now," complained Bob, a fifty-year-old director of a private elementary school. "I'm afraid they'll make me look...old."

"I'm pissed that I can't play ball like I used to. It messes up my back and the knee injury that I've lived with since high school slows me down too much," says Jeremy, a teacher at the local community college. "But if I don't exercise, I start getting a pot belly even when I eat well."

"I feel tired all the time," says George, a business consultant to Fortune 500 companies. "There's nothing wrong with me, but I don't have much energy and I have trouble sleeping at night."

"I'm losing it where it counts—in the sack," lamented Fred, a fifty-five-year-old rancher. "I've been married twice and things were pretty good up until recently. I just don't feel that turned on and sometimes I lose my erection when I need it the most. I even tried having an affair, but that only worked briefly and the problems returned. At first I blamed the problem on my wife. I tried to get her to be sexier and experiment more, but now I'm afraid it might be me and it scares me to death."

It seemed like we were all falling apart. All the bravado of youth seemed to have left us like air leaking out of a tire. Our lives were deflated. The only choices seemed to be to accept the downhill slide into oblivion and death or to deny the whole thing and go on with life as though nothing was happening. Most of us chose to ignore the whole thing. Others tried to reinvent their lost youth. "Maybe if I can find a fast car, a young woman, or a new life, I can keep from sliding down and stay on top of the mountain."

The bad news is that going down the mountain is inevitable. The good news is that there is another mountain on the other side. We can't really stay where we are or go back the way we came. We must move ahead if we are to continue to grow and mature as we age. The problem is that no one told us about the second mountain, so most of us are afraid to go down the first one, afraid that when we do, it will be the end.

Urgent, I'm Terrified

Until recently, male menopause was unheard of, a bar room joke. I hadn't associated myself with this issue until my therapist suggested I get your book. This is a particularly relevant issue in my life and I am experiencing many of the symptoms you list. I'm terrified that I will learn too late how to deal with this successfully and to effectively and happily finish the second half of my life.

Max

Points of understanding:

• For a long time, women's menopausal symptoms were not taken seriously. "It's all in her head, she's just being 'hysterical,' or looking for an excuse to be bitchy." We've viewed men in a similar way. "It's just a midlife crisis, he's just acting like a kid, or looking for an excuse to buy a sports car and find a trophy girlfriend." The truth is, menopause is probably the most significant life change a man or woman experiences in life. How a man or woman goes through this time will determine whether the next thirty, forty, or fifty years will be times of joy or despair.

• It's never too late to learn the skills you will need to move through this period effectively. It is uncharted territory. Use all the information you can find as a map that will bring you safely though it.

My Own Journey through the Male Menopause Passage

My first experience with male menopause occurred the day I was born on December 21, 1943. When my mother announced, "It's a boy," and lifted me up for my father to hold. He was thirty-seven years old and in the midst of a major life crisis. Over the next five years, he became increasingly depressed and withdrawn. He had what my mother called "a midlife nervous breakdown" and left before I was six. I grew up wondering what had happened to him. In some ways my whole life has been dedicated to understanding why he left and why so many other men leave at this time of life, through divorce, disease, despair, and death.

I was twenty-five years old when I held my own son moments after his birth. I vowed that I would be a different kind of father than my father had been for me. I had already been a practicing psychotherapist for a number of years, but with Jemal's birth I began to focus my professional interest on men's issues.

When I began going through male menopause I had no idea what was happening. I was in my forties, at the top of my profession, great kids, wonderful wife, good friends, a nice house in an upscale neighborhood. Everything was great. Yet, it seemed like my life was out of sync. At first there were small things, nothing I could put my finger on. I knew I felt irritable and angry a lot, but it all seemed the result of things that were going on "out there." Who wouldn't be angry if they had the boss I had, the money problems, the stresses at home, someone always wanting something. I felt like my world was out of balance but I didn't know why or what to do about it.

Emotionally, I seemed to be riding a rollercoaster. When I was "up" I wanted to work for days on end. My energy was endless and I gloried in the vision of taking life by the tail and swinging it wildly over my head. I was supremely confident that I could make a real difference in the world. But then the dark moods would come over me and I wanted to kill something, or at least beat the hell out of it.

"What" or "why" was a complete mystery to me. On the other side of anger was the depression, a beast I needed to keep at bay.

Though my wife Carlin and I were happy, it seemed that she wasn't as interested in me as she once was. "She seems to have time and energy for everyone else," I told myself. "I feel like I'm way down on her priority list." Our sex life was OK, but I worried about what it would be like in the future. I often felt hurt, then angry, then ashamed of being hurt and angry. I worried that we were drifting apart, but afraid to say anything about it. I felt like an insecure adolescent, but tried to hold it all in, tough it out, and wait for things to get better.

Things with my wife were good, yet I felt uneasy and confused. I had expected that when the kids were gone we would be closer, more intimate, and would finally have more time for each other, more time for sex. But within a week after our last child left home, Carlin went on a retreat and returned to announce she was starting a school—The Diamond-Wise School for Sacred Living and Joyful Action. She seemed on fire with passion, but it didn't seem directed at me.

Five-and-a-half years my senior, she had been going through menopause, a change neither one of us understood. For me it was a time of longing and disconnection. Just when I would be feeling close to Carlin, a hot flash would roar through her body like a wild fire in a forest and she would descend into an underworld where I could not follow and did not belong. I wanted to reach out and hold her and be held, but I wasn't sure she still wanted me.

At times I felt afraid to be in her presence. There was something overwhelming to me about her "post-menopausal zest." She had an "edge" about her that would cut into me when we would get close. I longed for more intimacy, but did not want to get hurt. Lovemaking was less frequent and less enjoyable. I was sure it was the beginning of the end of our sex lives. I even felt Carlin seemed happy enough to avoid sex altogether. I tried to be understanding but my mind kept screaming, "I'm too young to stop having sex." I thought about finding a younger partner but I loved my wife. I considered having an affair, but it seemed more fun in fantasy than reality. What I really wanted was my wife back.

It wasn't until after Carlin had gotten through her own menopause that I gradually suspected that I was going through mine. Letting the awareness in was not easy. Her changes were so much more dramatic that they easily eclipsed my own.

Looking at my career was a first step. My work was going well. I had been a therapist, author, workshop leader, and teacher for many years. Yet, I felt insecure there too. Even though I had worked hard to be good at what I did, I wondered whether there would come a time when all my clients would leave en masse, no one would buy any of my books or attend any of my classes, and I would have to start all over again. And even if it all went well I wasn't sure I wanted to spend another twenty, thirty, or forty years doing what I was doing. "When is my time going to come?" I wondered. "Is there more to life than this?"

The male menopause markers are only clear now in retrospect, like buoys that appear out of the fog.

I remember it was a Friday in July when Mom called complaining of chest pains. I told her I was on my way. My heart was beating fast, but I tried to remain calm as I drove from our house on the hill to the senior citizen complex where she lived. In the five minutes it took me to get there, thoughts and images cascaded through my mind: carrying boxes of household items up the stairs when she first arrived from southern California. Sitting on her deck surrounded by plants that she nurtured like children. Chuckling at the hand-lettered sign on her wall: "Senior Citizens: On Your Feet and Off Your Rockers." Smiling at the old records—*Harry Belafonte at the Hollywood Bowl, The Piano Artistry of Ferrante & Teicher, Percy Faith's Greatest Hits, Fiddler on the Roof.* And books, everywhere there were books, old ones and new ones, classics, romances, histories.

At the hospital she was examined by a doctor who didn't look old enough to be doing the job. He later announced that she was OK but wanted to have some X rays done. I felt relieved and told myself that there was never really anything to worry about. My Mom was still young, in her early seventies. Even though I was born when she was thirty-six, she always seemed young, vital, and engaged—more active doing volunteer work after she retired than she had been in her years as an executive secretary.

We were told she had an aneurysm that would have to be operated on. As we left the bright white busyness of the hospital, we talked for the first time about the possibility that she might die. I had a lump in my throat and tears that I was having trouble holding back. She seemed rather calm. "I'm not really afraid of death," she said looking straight ahead. "I've had a good life and I don't have many regrets. My only fear is that I would become disabled and be a burden on you and your family." I wanted to scream, "You're not a burden, you never could be a burden, you're my mother and I love you." But I didn't say anything. I didn't know how to put my feelings into words. The truth was I was scared, scared that she would die, scared that she would end up living with us and become a burden, scared I would turn out to be a lousy son who cared more about his own comfort than about what his aging mother needed. But all I could say was, "Oh, Mom, you're going to be just fine."

A friend asked me, "What are you going to do when your mother dies?" My response was immediate and angry. "What do you mean?" I nearly screamed. "You're talking like she's going to die." He was kind, but firm, "All our parents die sometime and we all need to prepare ourselves." I learned that his father had recently died and he was trying to pass on some wisdom that I resisted hearing.

Yet, over the weeks and months I couldn't get the thought of death out of my mind. During the day, I would stay busy with work, but at night, it would creep in around the edges of my consciousness, grab a hold of my mind when I least expected it. I remembered my friend Gary who had died the year before. It was a shock to everyone. He was only forty. The death certificate said the cause of death was the result of an auto accident. Those of us who knew him well believed that the real cause was his excessive drinking, his compulsive sexual behavior that was threatening to end his marriage, and his depression that he refused to confront.

I didn't want to think about these things or open up to the feelings that the thoughts demanded. So, I did what I had always done when I was uncomfortable with feelings. I plunged more fully into my job. Work was always a place I could go to escape from things I didn't want to confront. But, like most men, I never thought of it as an escape. It was just something I did. I could feel good that I was working for my family, or to make the world a little better place, or to make enough money to buy the things we needed and wanted. Work was always there. It was like a wife, a lover, a friend.

I remember one of those midlife evenings when I was able to talk openly with my wife about how we felt about our past "loves." She talked about the relationship with her first boyfriend, with girlfriends in college, with people she was close to now. She wanted to know who were the loves in my life. Of course, I said that she was. She expected to hear that and I really felt it. But in looking back I realized that for me my most passionate relationships had been with jobs I had held.

I remembered selling Christmas cards to neighbors when I was seven years old, my first paperback route when I was nine, selling magazines when I was ten and again when I was nineteen. I worked for a division of the United Nations when I was sixteen. During summers in college, I worked in hospitals. Later, I worked in various health clinics.

Each memory was sharp, clear, and luminous. As my wife talked about her "loves" and I talked about "my work," I realized they each elicited similar feelings. There were those we loved unconditionally, some we hated but stayed with. Most we had mixed feelings towards. But work, which had always been a faithful, though often difficult, companion was beginning to change. In the past when I got restless, which I did every few years, there always seemed to be a new job waiting for me.

Things were different now. I wasn't sure I wanted another job to find me or for me to find another job. I thought I might like to do something completely different from anything I had ever done. I had fantasies about quitting everything and taking a trip across country. My wife encouraged me and we decided that a break from the day-to-day grind might make everything better. We took off and did some traveling, but that didn't seem to solve things.

Instead of a carefree vacation, we fought all along our route. I felt that everything she did was an irritation to me. I knew that she wasn't to blame for my unhappiness, but I couldn't get past the feeling that it was somehow her fault that things weren't better in our lives. "If only she'd…"—there seemed to be no end to what I would put in the blank. "If only she'd be more interested in sex…be more caring…be more appreciative of how hard I work."

On one level, the trip was a disaster; on another, it was a triumph. I remember places across the U.S. in connection with how big a fight we had just before, during, or after we were there. The first eruption occurred prophetically in Volcano, California, and continued through Elko, Nevada; Green River, Utah; Boulder, Colorado; and on across the heartland of America. The last one occurred just outside Ann Arbor, Michigan, when I got so mad I got out of the camper and slammed the door so hard I shattered the window on the driver's side of the vehicle. A rage was eating me up inside. I had no idea where it was coming from, but it seemed to have been stalking me for a long time. I felt I needed to kill it before I hurt someone.

It felt like the only way I could keep from hurting myself, my wife, or both of us was to get away. My wife was terrified of my outburst, but wanted to stay and talk it out. I finally left amid her tears and said I'd meet her in a week at my uncle and aunt's house in Florida.

I was scared, but also exhilarated. I felt free again, free like I remembered feeling when I went to Europe when I was twenty. I knew it wasn't my wife I was mad at, but I also knew that I couldn't fight the demons that were beginning to rage within me without putting her in danger. Though I didn't know it at the time, the only way to show her my love and protect her from harm was to get away from her.

I've found this is true for many men. We are often accused of being unfeeling and insensitive when in fact we are sometimes too sensitive. We are afraid to let out the anger that smolders inside. Over the years, the pressure builds up and turns into rage which terrifies us. Finally, like men in wars who would fall on a live grenade to protect their buddies, men trap their rage inside to protect those around them. The result is the depression and increased suicide rate we see with men as they move past forty.

I've learned other, hopefully more compassionate, ways to show love and protect my wife and children since then. But for many men and the women they live with, the burning anger men feel is a complete mystery.

Anger and depression also are tied to the physical and sexual problems that men must confront as we age. Many men begin having heart problems, high blood pressure, prostate problems, diabetes, and sexual difficulties. These problems often feed on each other. When we're depressed, we lose our desire and ability to make love. When we're having erection problems, we easily become more depressed. Without outside help, the downward spiral keeps us caught in the undertow.

Like so many men, I couldn't admit I was depressed. My wife would say I seemed down, irritated, and worried. She would call it my "beady-eyed" look. When she'd ask how I was, I would say I was "fine." I didn't really feel fine, but I couldn't say how I felt. It just seemed that I had slipped into a fog that was now so familiar I just felt "fine." Fine, for me, was more like same as usual, not good, not horrible, just blah.

The more she'd ask about me, the more irritated I would get. "Just leave me alone," I'd yell. Or else, I'd just keep my mouth shut and let the feelings fester inside. It just hurt too much and was too confusing to try and figure out what was really going on with me. It seemed so much easier to stay numb most of the time with periodic angry outbursts at something she did or didn't do.

I was hungry to feel her love and be close. I felt desperate. In my desperation, I would get angry and push Carlin away even more. The more she withdrew, the more fearful I became and the more desperate to reconnect. It was a horrible spiral that was taking us both down and one that neither of us could break on our own.

One of the greatest gifts I received from my wife was her willingness to hang in there and not give up on me or our marriage. I finally read a book that told me the same things she had been telling me for years. I went to a doctor, who did a complete mental and physical exam, and diagnosed depression. She recommended a combination of medications and cognitive behavior therapy. It was as though years of frozen ice began to break up, not all at once, but a little at a time. I knew things were going to get better and I would survive my change of life with my marriage intact.

The Struggle Is Worth It: Helen and Roy's Story

After reading your book, Roy and I got into counseling. It had taken years. Roy had said all along that he didn't need counseling. Even when our marriage was in shambles, he insisted we needed to work things out ourselves. When I finally called and you talked to us both, Roy finally understood the benefits that counseling could provide.

I am not sure if the counseling is doing very much for me but it seems to be helping Roy a lot so I will continue with it. I find myself arguing a lot with this therapist because he doesn't take the male menopause issue as seriously as he should.

I had to bring the book in and show him a thing or two and then I explained why I know it relates to Roy. Then he listened a little more. He has given Roy some very good advice that is working for him. He asked Roy what his goal was in doing counseling. Roy told him it was to keep his wife and hang on to his marriage. Whenever he has thoughts that make him want to act in certain ways, he encourages Roy to remember his goal. If whatever it is does not do something to get to that goal he should *not do it today*.

It seems to help a lot. Today, Roy told me that he uses this at least once each day. (I didn't realize how much of a struggle this still is for him.) And I have been just trying to support him as much as I can. I try to constantly show him how important he is to me and how much I want us to stay married. I kiss him every day like there is no tomorrow and actually the intimate part of our relationship seems to be better than ever before.

Roy says this every time we go to counseling and I agree. I have faith that we will make it through this, although it does not seem that way most of the time. You told me not to give up and when I start to feel like it is too much, I remember those encouraging words.

It is only just recently (the past few days) that I am starting to be able to push away the thoughts that come to mind and haunt my days and nights. It drives me crazy to remember that he had a relationship with a twenty-three-year-old girl, and that he was actually going to leave me. These things, as well as Roy's depression, are the hardest things to handle. But we are beginning to deal with this a little better now. I know you encouraged me to get counseling for myself and get into a woman's group. I may do that in the future, but I guess I'm not ready yet.

We are still working on these issues that have come between us. He has a lot of other issues that I was unaware of and that he has stuffed inside and ignored for so long that he doesn't feel he can blame his actions on the male menopause. I feel differently. I feel like your book *Male Menopause* was written about *him*. But I also remember that you told us the severity of the symptoms depended on many factors including past life experiences.

I don't know if I mentioned that my husband is a "son of a preacher" (as he refers to it). He was raised so strictly that it was almost abusive. Roy is just now beginning to recognize how much hurt and shame he stuffed inside when he was growing up. His older brother was always favored and Roy was told that he would never amount to anything, that he was just a "Mama's boy."

When he would disobey his father, he was made to go outside and find a switch. If it wasn't big enough he had to go back until he found one that was the right size. He then had to pull down his pants and was beaten until he bled.

I cried when he brought this out in counseling. I had no idea that had happened to him when he was a child. Even with support, Roy didn't want to talk about it for a long time and when he did he couldn't let his feelings out. Now he's beginning to let out some of the anger. It's very painful, but he is hanging in there with it, though he threatens to quit every week.

Since we began counseling, Roy has become more loving and less angry. He's started to talk more. We seem to have broken the stony silences that were the norm in our relationship for so long. He's even smiling again. His face was always scowling. I thought it would just freeze that way. But now the ice seems to be melting.

He has started doing things that he had once enjoyed, but had long abandoned. He wants to go out again. We've even been to some parties which we had stopped going to years ago. Roy has also developed some new interests. He's learned how to tat and is making lace for our daughter's upcoming wedding. He says it relaxes him. He still gets upset at times, but he seems much more open to listening to me and letting me give him some loving support.

I keep telling him to remember his goal when he gets discouraged and to keep working on healing. As you told us, if we don't heal the old wounds, they come back to haunt us. Since listening to Roy, I realize that I grew up in a very similar kind of family. My father was very strict with my brothers and very sweet to me. He was a perfect father until I began to go through puberty. As soon as my body began to change, he withdrew from me. When he did relate to me, it was to criticize what I was wearing or how I looked. I could never understand what changed for him. Now I'm beginning to recognize that he was going through male menopause and having a lot of the symptoms I've been seeing in Roy.

It seems the things that come from our upbringing can certainly make male menopause a huge issue. We have learned a great deal. We still have a very long way to go. I do however see a big change in my husband for the better. He has taken a very clear look at what he has in this marriage and he is very glad that I have stayed with him through all this. It is still very hard but I feel we are getting closer.

Helen

Going through Male Menopause Together: Linda and Jake's Story

Linda had read the Dear Abby column and called with the familiar story that her husband, Jake, seemed to be experiencing all the symptoms I mentioned but refused to get help.

Dear Jed,

I called and talked to you when I saw your Dear Abby that was printed in an Ohio newspaper about the symptoms of male menopause. We are having such an incredible struggle. My biggest concern is for my husband's depression. It is so bad. We found a doctor that specializes in hormones but NOT male menopause. He is very understanding. You told me about your book, *Male Menopause,* and I read it and so did my husband. We gave it to our doctor and he said he would read it. Then we went out and bought your new revised paperback. I found it so interesting. As I read, I underlined things that pertained to my husband. Then my husband did the same. We were amazed at how much this book talked about my husband.

I know him well and I know he is having a hard time. Very hard. Is there anything else I can do to help him through this depression until the medicine starts to work? We also are seeing our pastor and are getting professional counseling. Nothing is helping him to feel better. All of his hormone levels are "normal" according to the doctor but the doctor will not take a total testosterone test. Please tell me what I can do to help my husband or tell me where to find help for him. I really worry about this depression because it brings him down so much. My husband has always taken good care of himself and watches what he eats. We also belong to a health club where we go work out almost every day. He takes more vitamins than anyone I know. He always has. But what else can we do? This is so hard!

Linda

I sent another letter of encouragement and gave Linda some more suggestions. Two weeks later, I got her hopeful reply.

Jed,

Thank you for the quick reply to my email message. We have found a psychologist that we think could be helpful. We will have our second and third visit this week with him. In the meantime, my husband's new dose of Prozac seems to be working. Of course, we read and heard on The Learning Channel just this week that Prozac could effect his sex drive so that is a big drawback for a man going through this male menopause. But at least we know and can do something about it if it does effect him in that way. So I think we are headed in the right direction.

I just wanted to thank you for your reply and to let you know that if it wasn't for the article someone sent me from that Ohio newspaper, my husband and I would have had no idea about real male menopause and he would have (without a doubt) moved out by now and would have been drinking himself into the hospital (he has a condition that he is not to have alcohol) and he would have been with the girl he was seeing (seventeen years younger than me). And there is a good chance that I may have followed through with some of the suicide thoughts I was having because I had such a hard time when I found out my husband had been with someone else.

The love we have between us has always been something so special and so different than most couples. I could not see life without him. It is because of you and the information you gave me on the phone, in your books, and even in your email that my husband is still here today and that we are working through this. He is finally feeling better and I feel he is now more able to get something from our counseling.

Thanks again. As you counseled, I will never give up. My husband is definitely worth the work involved.

It's Hard to Talk about My Feelings: Jake's Story

Jake's telling of his story touches on many of the common feelings visited throughout the male menopausal years. His response is a rare glimpse into the inner working of the male mind at this stage of life.

Talking about myself has been very difficult and counseling was the last thing I thought I needed. I don't think I would have considered it if Linda hadn't insisted. I knew I didn't want to lose my marriage and I was willing to try anything.

I don't know what's scientifically common or uncommon. I do know what everyone on the planet thinks about men, myself included. When I look at myself I see a male of the human species that from puberty on has had mainly one thing on his mind—sex.

Of course, there are many things of other concern that interfere by necessity, like eating and housing and work. But at any given moment of any day it would seem that if it's not slapping me right in the face, then sex is at least in some form of underlying thought or idea.

Is that a "male" attitude? Or is it just me? It's my opinion, from working around men all my life, that it's every male in the world to a greater or lesser degree.

That's where these last few years or so of my life come into focus. Or should I say into blur? There was a change in my thoughts. My feelings about myself and about my sexuality began to change. I didn't notice it as a change at the time, but I notice it now as I look back. And even now I probably wouldn't have noticed it if my wife hadn't pointed things out.

Some of the changes were fundamental. I remember hearing people talk about depression—my sister, my wife, strangers in the newspaper. I heard stories of how it would push them into committing desperate acts. It had always been this distant, abstract idea of a thing that I could not understand.

When I had problems, I'd just say to myself, "It's all in your head. Just get it out of there." What in the world could anyone get so down about that they could actually take their own life? Or how could they yell at their wives, leave their families, lose their passion for life, look for a younger woman, or do many of the other things that people do when they are depressed?

I can honestly say I didn't have two minutes of depression in my entire life until three years ago. I can now understand what depression really is. Not since I was a child did I feel such a deep-seated anger and sadness. I would yell and I would cry. I couldn't believe it was me. Here I was, a forty-five-year-old grown man, a truck driver, for heaven's sake, throwing a tantrum like a four-year-old or bawling like a baby.

Looking back now I can see that the depression preceded the affair I had with a younger woman by two years, though at the time I didn't feel depressed. It felt more like everyone else went out of their way to irritate me. I loved my wife, but the passion seemed to be draining out of our relationship. I didn't realize it was really the passion draining out of me.

My thinking began to change. I wasn't getting enough of what I needed, but I didn't know how to ask for what was important to me. I felt like my manhood was slipping away and I didn't know what to do.

That was when I started noticing the twenty-eight-year-old waitress who began to work at one of the restaurants I often stopped at when I was on the road driving. She was interested in me. She found me attractive. I felt complimented. I felt wanted. At that time, my wife and I were doing well together but we had come through some hard times with my kids living with us two years before. I think I carried some bitterness toward her and my kids for a situation that I didn't seem to have any control over. It's awful to feel powerless over a situation.

I sure felt like it would be so wonderful to get out from under all these responsibilities. With my new girl, I felt young and capable and powerful again. I think I knew my wife still loved me and wanted me, but there was so much baggage.

Or maybe it was the bitterness, a form of discontent caused by unresolved anger and doubt.

So I had a chance for something that I thought I would never have a chance at again. How many guys pushing fifty would in their wildest dreams have a girl that young and attractive come after them?

I took it. I know now that I absolutely should not have. What a high price to pay, to risk the loss of my marriage, for such a short-lived pleasure. But it ended as quickly as it started. And the truth is I honestly did love my wife. We both tried to forget about the affair and get on with our lives. "Let the past stay frozen where it is and make the present flow," I thought. It seemed that things returned to normal and my wife and I we were getting along fine.

Yet, I still felt a deep discontent. The depression came back, light gage at first, but got worse as time went on. I started having a hard time with details. I was working on remodeling the attic and couldn't seem to do the job right. I was impatient and wouldn't take the time to read the directions and do the measurements correctly. It just became too much for me. The project still remains, to this day, unfinished. It was just one more thing that wasn't like me. I'd always considered myself somewhat of a perfectionist and prided myself on my ability to complete things ahead of schedule. I just felt like I had to escape.

It also bled into other aspects of my emotional life. Though I wasn't even sure I had an emotional life. Things were either good or bad and why bother thinking about anything bad?

"Everything is just fine," I would tell myself. "Things will always take care of themselves, and if for some reason they don't, then I'll handle it. Who cares?" I wish I still had that positive attitude and confidence. My wife calls it cockiness. I seem to have lost that some-how. It has been replaced by worry, reluctance, and doubt.

That was another thing I found that drew me to the younger woman. She gave me a renewed sense of power, a clear sense of direction. She made me feel strong and important. I felt important. We were important to each other. I felt needed again. She often made the comment, "We're so good together." That's something that over time seems to get unintentionally swept under the carpet with your spouse.

With my spouse I often felt awkward, like two teenagers who don't know how to kiss and bump noses and arms. I felt like we were walking on eggshells, afraid to make the wrong move. I felt like I couldn't do anything right, that as a man I was a complete klutz, if not a failure. I never felt that with the younger woman.

I never knew that depression in men often expresses itself in anger. That was certainly the case with me. I was often irritated and grouchy and sometimes would have angry outbursts over the least little thing. That is so totally unlike me, I tended to blame it on my wife. I've always had an easygoing, calm, and happy personality.

One of the most difficult aspects of this time of life is the uncer-tainty. I question everything. I have faith in nothing. Even though I hate the way I feel, I can't seem to help it. Again, you would have to know me to know the immensity of those statements. Explainable or not, that is truly how I feel right now.

To make a long story short, my wife's detective work and my sloppy sneaking around brought my three-month affair to an end. She had bought your book searching for some explanation for my behavior. Let me tell you, Jed, I read it after her and she had underlined in pencil what she thought pertained to us. The end result was that there was hardly a page without many underlinings. You could have titled that book, *The Life and Recent Times of Jake*.

There is one thing I would like to say to others, one bit of advice that is totally out of a man's control, which is the way one's wife handles the crisis. In my case, I was as fortunate as I could possibly be in this. I can see things in my wife now that I have been blind to for the past fourteen years. It's amazing to me that I could close my eyes and refuse to see the obvious for so long. In the end, some years from now, whichever way this story goes, I will never doubt that my wife *really* loved me. She has dealt with her deep heartache without making me feel even worse than I do.

She has tried in every way possible to help me get through this mysterious emotional passage. I know now how devastating my affair was to my wife and to our marriage. When a marriage suffers such a potentially deadly blow, and when the one who took that blow turns their attention to the healing of their attacker, I think it can only be real love at work.

Jake

Points of understanding:

• It's very difficult for men to recognize their deepest feelings. Expressing them to someone else is even more difficult. Yet, with enough support and understanding men are hungry to be heard. Jake is a wonderful example of a man who has taken the opportunity to share his feelings and tell his story.

• Counseling can be very helpful to men as a support outside the family. Yet, counseling is foreign territory for most men. It can be greatly beneficial when they do it, but they resist it like crazy at first.

• Sex, though complex, is nearly a constant presence in the minds of most men between puberty and male menopause. We know that testosterone in men fluctuates three to four times an hour, which may account for the reports that men think about sex nearly constantly. It's a huge change when sexuality begins to shift at midlife.

• For most men, the changes are subtle at first—injuries take longer to heal, joints are more stiff, we tire more easily, and become irritable more quickly. It is often the women in our lives that first notice the changes, which is why it is so important for women to understand male menopause and know what to do to be helpful. (It's also important for men to understand menopause in women, a job we haven't done very well in the past.)

• Depression in men is quite common during this period, even for those who couldn't imagine it happening to them. This is not just in a man's head. Though there are emotional changes that men experience, there are also significant hormonal and physical changes that can shake the very foundations of a man's world.

• Anger and sadness are often constant companions and a man is thrown from one to the other. He feels helpless and out of control. For men who have been in control most of their lives, this is a particularly difficult time. Understanding the process and having a "road map" through to the other side can be tremendously helpful.

• Although an affair, either in thought or deed, is often a dramatic marker of this change for many men, it usually comes many years after other symptoms of male menopause, such as depression. This is why these early warning signs are so important to notice, so we can avoid more serious problems later.

• Many will say, "I love you, but I'm not in love with you." What they really mean is that it seems that the passion is draining out of the relationship. Many men (and women) say it feels more like they are living with a roommate than a lover. Men often blame their spouse. Jake's line says it clearly and should be emblazoned on the headboards of every bed in the world, "I didn't realize it was really the passion draining out of me." If men and women understood this, it would save millions from divorce and heartbreak.

• Men know something is wrong. We often look outside ourselves for what is missing and feel that "you aren't giving me what I need." We often aren't even sure what it is that we need, how to ask for it if we did know, or how to accept what is given if we got it. We feel more and more impoverished, and in our panic it feels that we are losing the core of our being, that our manhood is slipping away.

• It's no wonder that men feel particularly drawn to women who might fill the void that is opening up inside them. As Jake says, "She was interested in me. She found me attractive. I felt complimented. I felt wanted." Many men don't realize that what is missing cannot be filled by a woman, it must be filled from within. Yet, it's difficult to say no when the opportunity arises.

• Men feel powerless over so many things at this time of life. Our bodies are changing, our hormones are fluctuating, our parents are getting sick and dying, our children are growing up and leaving, our mates are going through their own changes, our jobs can't be counted on to sustain us. We look for something to hold on to. In our confused mind, we think, "Maybe a twenty-eight-year-old waitress is what I need."

• Life at home seems so weighty, so complicated. The baggage from the past seems too much to handle. We dream of chucking it all and running off to…Alaska? A new job? A new woman? An endless sleep? A spiritual adventure?

• Men often jump ship and regret it later. They find that none of the escapes really give them what they are missing. They long to come home, or they stay in between. They can't seem to leave, but they don't want to stay. If they can work out the conflicts, their marriage and family life can become even stronger.

• The first step is to recognize that escape does not work, that we have to face our feelings, no matter how painful they are, and deal honestly with our emotional life, which we kept hidden for so long.

• Men lose their confidence during this time. They worry more and are plagued by doubt. They have lost the map to their lives. The steering mechanism of their ship malfunctions and they flounder. It's a terrifying experience. They need support in understanding that this is preparing them for a more secure future, not the end of the world.

• Jake's words about his relationship with Linda need to be highlighted. They help us understand a great deal about this period. We feel awkward with our partner, it's easy to begin to drift away to a safer distance. Other women become interesting because they don't see our foibles and we can pretend confidence we don't really feel.

• For men, depression often expresses itself as irritation and anger. We don't seem sad, but angry. We believe the anger is justified and that everyone, particularly our spouse, is going out of her way to hurt us. "Who wouldn't be angry when she does that stuff?" Helping a man recognize his depression is a crucial part of recovery at this stage of life.

• Since everything seems so uncertain and changeable, a man grasps for things he can count on. He's afraid of what's ahead, so he clings to the past. He denies that anything is wrong in the mistaken belief that pretending nothing is wrong will make everything OK.

• Most spouses want desperately to help their partners, but don't know how. Understanding and compassion will be tested like never before. Initially, most men will resent their wives' concern and will see it as meddling. He will often push her away, emotionally and sometimes physically. Learning to protect yourself from abuse, while keeping your vision focused on the kind of relationship you want is one of the greatest challenges a person will face in their life.

• Jake's words are a tribute to a wife who stuck it out and a man who was willing to recognize and acknowledge the pain he had caused: "When a marriage suffers such a potentially deadly blow, and when the one who took that blow turns their attention to the healing of their attacker, I think it can only be real love at work."

***

In future chapters you will hear from other women and men about what they have experienced. You will come to understand male menopause as a natural, yet very misunderstood and difficult life transition. With this information, you will be in a much better position to help your own relationships succeed.

Chapter 2

Everything You Always Wanted to Ask about Male Menopause, But Were Afraid to Know

"Gee, I hope there's such a thing as male menopause. Because if there isn't...what *was* that." Dave Fishberg, a sixty-year-old songwriter and piano player speaks for many men I have talked to about this vital change in their lives. We often only understand who we are after we have moved to another phase of the life cycle.

One way to think of male menopause is like puberty in reverse. How many of us understood who we were when we were in the middle of being a teenager? I believe male menopause is one of the most important, yet least understood, periods of a man's life.

Male menopause is more than a midlife crisis because it involves the body, mind, and spirit, and goes to the very heart of what it means to be a man in the second half of life.

It's interesting that two of our youngest presidents, Kennedy and Clinton, went through this period of life in the spotlight of public attention, and it seems clear that both these men had real difficulty.

The First Family is unique only because so much public attention is focused on them. But I have been seeing similar crises in families all over the country and around the world. The question I hear over and over is, Why do midlife men do such dumb things?

Remember that great song from the 1960s by Buffalo Springfield? There was a lyric that sticks in my mind. "Something's happening here, what it is ain't exactly clear." That's how I began to feel as a therapist when I saw so many men experiencing problems at this time of life.

What Exactly Is Male Menopause?

Male menopause (also called viropause or andropause) is a multidimensional change of life with hormonal, physical, psychological, interpersonal, sexual, and spiritual aspects. All aspects are equally important and all must be understood and treated. They are all present with men during this period of time, though they may not all be of equal intensity or equally obvious.

Tired Most of the Time, Self-Confidence Is Nil

I have just discovered your website, and was referred to it by a friend who knows the man I live with. He is forty-eight years old and has been getting more and more frustrated with his lack of response to psychotherapy, antidepressants, etc. He has been through all of it, up to and including wondering if he might be ADD, and taking medication for that, just in case it might help. It didn't.

He feels tired most of the time (even though he takes vitamins and works out at the gym with weights and on the treadmill at least three times a week), has trouble sleeping, and is becoming more and more depressed with time. With the latest bout of severe depression has come anxiety, a new and unwelcome development. He has difficulty concentrating and remembering things (hence the tests for ADD), he can't decide what to do with his life, he has decreasing amounts of self-confidence (now down to about nil), and he is nearly too consumed by fear to make any kind of decision.

Although I try to be understanding, he seems extremely irritable and we fight more than we ever have.

Whether due to the depression, antidepression medication, or male menopause (we haven't discussed the reason), there has been no interest in sex for many months. I'm desperate to understand what is going on.

Louise

Point of understanding:

Louise's description of her husband's male menopause experience emphasizes the physical, psychological, interpersonal, and sexual dimensions.

Libido Is Low But Finds Joy Mentoring Young Men

I'm a fifty-five-year-old man who has been working all of his life. I've been married twice and have one grown daughter. For most of my life I felt like I ran the show. I've started a number of companies, made a lot of money, and lost a lot of money.

The thing that's bothering me the most now is that I feel like I've lost my libido. It isn't just that I don't feel sexual, but it feels that my whole life energy is down. My mind is active, but my spirit is low.

I've been retired for a number of years and it felt good to kick back and take a rest after working my whole life. But six months ago, two events changed my life. The first was when I decided to apply to be a mentor with Big Brothers/Big Sisters. I was assigned a ten-year-old boy, an only child whose father had deserted the mother when the boy was six. We've become great pals and I find it very satisfying to teach him things and just to spend time together.

I've also met with other Big and Little Brothers. It touches something very deep in me. I'm able to give the boys some of the fathering I never got. I also feel I'm making a difference in the world, contributing to something bigger than myself. I feel like I want to do more. I almost feel called to do more. But I'm not sure if it's just my ego. I'm also not sure if I have the energy to do more.

The other major happening occurred when I called an old friend in California whom I had known many years ago. She had been my banker at one time and I needed some advice on some investments I was considering. She invited me out for a visit and we quickly fell in love.

At first, things were fine, though sexually it took some time to feel comfortable with each other. I can get erections OK, though they're not as hard as they were when I was younger, but I don't feel a whole lot of sexual energy between us. I love her, I love the way her body looks. I just don't feel much of a turn-on.

I went to the doctor and had my testosterone levels checked. He told me I was in the low to normal range and I might want to consider testosterone replacement therapy. What do you think? Could testosterone help restore my vitality and desire?

Kevin

Point of understanding:

The hormonal, social, and spiritual dimensions are prominent with this man, though sexual, psychological, interpersonal, and physical aspects are also present. It's really impossible to separate one dimension from the others. They are all interrelated.

He Doesn't Have Any Interest in Women, Not Even Me

I love a wonderful man that for no "real" reason, left after our being together for several years. He just fits the image you write about so perfectly. At forty-three years of age, he did a total turn around, becoming selfish, angry, forgetful, and indecisive. He says he still cares about me, but needs to find himself. The worst part is

that he does not have any interest in women, not even me. He won't see a doctor. He says that nothing is wrong with him. What can I do?
Sally

Points of understanding:

• Many men and women feel that male menopause isn't real, that a man's actions seem to be totally mysterious. Yet, becoming self-centered, angry, forgetful, and indecisive are some of the most common symptoms of male menopause.

• Some men become obsessed with women, others lose all interest.

• Most men deny that anything is wrong and refuse to seek help. There are ways to get through to them.

• Learning about male menopause is the first step in the process.

What Are the Most Common Signs of Male Menopause?

Hormonal: Drop in testosterone, free testosterone, DHEA, melatonin, thyroid hormone, and others.

Physical: Increased fatigue, short-term memory loss, persistent weight gain.

Psychological: Irritability, indecisiveness, and depression.

Interpersonal: A longing for intimacy and fear of getting close.

Social: Desire for close friendships and recognition of social isolation.

Sexual: Lowering of sexual desire, erectile dysfunctions, and fears of sexual loss.

Spiritual: Great restlessness and a longing to follow soul's calling.

Although all men go through male menopause and will experience some or all of these signs at some time during their midlife, they are not all equally common. Male menopause, as a field of research, is where female menopause was forty years ago.

Dr. Malcolm Carruthers, a specialist in treating male menopause, has been carrying out research for the past twenty years on the changes men go through during this stage of their lives. He has now completed a study of two thousand men going through male menopause. He presented his findings at the Second World Congress on the Aging Male held in Geneva, Switzerland, February 2000. His research findings need to be understood by men and women going through this change of life, as well as the medical profession who must become partners in treating them.

A Simple Cry For Help

Hi, I'm forty-five years old and have all the symptoms you describe as male menopause—sex, depression, physical problems. You name it, I've got it. What can I do? Can you help me?

Ronald

Points of understanding:

• This letter represents the hundreds I have received from men around the country and throughout the world. Most are short, direct, and to the point. There is little about the men and the details of their lives, feelings, or fears. It's almost as if they were saying, "I've got a bad cough. Give me a pill to make it go away so I can get back to work, quick."

• Men need to learn that male menopause is much more interesting and complex than a bad cough. But we need to start where men are and give them what they are asking for. Then we can help them deal with the deeper aspects of male menopause.

How Common Are the Symptoms of Male Menopause?

Men in Dr. Carruthers' study ranged in age from thirty-one to eighty, the mean being fifty-four.

• Reduced libido or sex drive was present in 80 percent of the men.

• Reduced potency or ability to obtain and maintain an erection was present in 80 percent of the men.

• Fatigue or loss of vitality was present in 80 percent of the men.

• Depression was present in 70 percent of the men.

• Aches, pains, and stiffness were reported by 65 percent of the men.

• Irritability and anger were present in 60 percent of the men. (My own findings indicate that this figure is much higher for men in the U.S., perhaps as high as 80 percent or 90 percent.)

• Night sweats were experienced by 50 percent of the men.

• Dryness and thinning of the skin was present in 46 percent of the men.

• Hot flashes were experienced by 25 percent of the men.

• Premature ejaculation and delayed ejaculation were present in 25 percent of the men.

• Stress was experienced by 60 percent of the men. (My own findings indicate that men in the U.S. report levels that are around 80 percent.)

• Excessive alcohol use was present in 35 percent of the men.

• Medications that interfere with potency were present in 30 percent of the men.

• Injuries and operations that interfere with potency, including vasectomy, were present in 30 percent of the men. (I suspect that circumcision causes similar problems.)

• Infections such as mumps, smoking, and obesity were present in 20 percent of the men.

What Is the Purpose of Male Menopause?

The purpose of male menopause is to signal the end of the first part of a man's life and prepare him for the second half. Male menopause is not the beginning of the end, as many fear, but the end of the beginning. It is the passage to the most passionate, powerful, productive, and purposeful time of a man's life.

How Long Does Male Menopause Last?

Male menopause generally takes five to fifteen years to complete. How long it takes depends on many factors. Remember, this is not simply a psychological shift from one stage of life to another, but involves all seven dimensions. We don't go from adolescence to adulthood overnight. The change from first adulthood to second adulthood can take as long or longer than moving through puberty.

It also depends on how tightly we cling to first adulthood. Many men have a fanatical desire to stay forever young. They associate becoming older with becoming frail, sexless, and lifeless. The more we cling to the past, the longer it takes to embrace the future. The journey is inevitable. We can no more resist male menopause than we can resist puberty. We can fight it, but we can't avoid it. Inevitably, we must move through it to the other side.

So Close to Cashing It All In

I can't even begin to describe how deeply your book has hit home for me in so many ways, on so many levels, with so many tears. I could write a book about how much this brought up for me—shame, abuse, absent father, male battering, and on and on. At this time of my life I've had to re-look at everything. I feel that men have been programmed, I have been programmed, to be protectors and often socially conditioned to be disposable.

I long to do something big in my life. Something that is meaningful. There is so much this planet needs to keep humans from destroying themselves and I yearn to do something helpful. It is not a selfish, egocentric, fear-based wish. It is an unfathomable gut-wrenching, heart-burning, throat-constricting, soul-shaking, unfilled yearning. Words cannot convey its depth. It is there. It always has been.

I'm so close to cashing it all in. I'm so fucking close. I'm frozen in my confusion and pain. I feel so ashamed to even be letting you in on my dilemma—your life has to be so hectic and you've already given so much of yourself. Your perspective is so unique, you've hit me so close to home. I just need to know that I'm not crazy and that someone else is struggling with these issues.

Carl

Points of understanding:

• Male menopause is truly a time of descending into the depth of our being. It is terrifying, particularly if we don't have a guide. One of the purposes of this book is to give women and men the support they need to begin this inward journey.

• At this stage of life, men and women often realize how much we have allowed society to program us to fulfill roles that limit and restrict us.

• Men have been programmed to "play hurt," suffer in silence, always be the protector, put our lives on the line, and "go down with the ship."

• Male menopause is a time that we confront our roles and hopefully commit to change in the future. It is a time when men want to do something big, something beyond themselves and their families. Men become more community focused and long to make a difference in the world. If this energy does not find expression, they settle for lesser goals like trading in their wife for a younger woman. Depression, despair, and, too often, suicide result when men aren't able to give to their full potential. The key issue for men at this time is to know that they are not crazy, that they are not alone, and that they can be helped.

How Many Men Are Going Through Male Menopause?

• In the U.S., there are 25,172,000 men between the ages of forty and fifty-five who are now going through male menopause.

• By 2020, the number of men in the U.S. going through male menopause will grow to approximately 57,500,000.

• Worldwide, there are approximately 408 million men between the ages of forty and fifty-five who are going through male menopause.

• By 2020, the number will grow to approximately 690 million men worldwide.

How Does Male Menopause Differ from Midlife Crisis and Aging?

Until recently, it has been assumed that the "change of life" for men was primarily psychological, while the change for women was primarily hormonal. The "midlife" crisis was therefore seen as a psychological and perhaps spiritual disruption where men went off the deep end and did crazy things. This midlife transition does not have to be a crisis. It only becomes one when we overemphasize the psychological dimension, attempt to ignore the other aspects of the "change," or try to deny the process altogether.

Aging is the effect of any energy flow on matter over time. It is inevitable and continues until we die. Time leads to the gradual accumulation of waste products and damage that eventually wears out the body, even in the absence of disease. Aging goes on forever. Male menopause is a time-limited transition period.

What Effect Are the Baby Boomers Having on Male Menopause?

The seventy-six million baby boomers in the U.S. born between 1946 and 1964 are changing the way everyone views midlife and aging. They are the first to recognize the importance of male menopause and they continue to have a profound influence on the culture. Baby boomers and their children now comprise about 50 percent of the U.S. population. They control an estimated 55 percent of consumer spending, head roughly 44 percent of the households, and make up most of the electorate. Better educated than any previous generation, they are the first to understand the importance of the mind/body connection in moving through menopause.

Why Haven't We Heard More about Male Menopause?

Men respond to their hormone rhythms in a way that reflects their culturally acquired self-image. They deny them. For a man, going through this time of life is frightening. He may already feel like he is losing it, that his manhood is deserting him. Admitting that his changes may be hormonal as much as psychological may raise more fears.

This denial extends to the largely male scientific and medical communities and accounts for why it has taken so long to study male menopause in more depth. Men who are out of touch with their body rhythms, afraid that "cycles" are feminine and hence to be avoided at all costs, are unlikely to be aware of the whisperings within until they get very loud.

Why Is It Important to Recognize Male Menopause Early On?

Every relationship is different and the consequences of a delayed diagnosis will vary from couple to couple. However, anytime there is a block to communication or a denial of personal, physical, or spiritual problems, the strength of a relationship will lessen. Keep your eyes open to what is going on in your relationship and speak honestly to one another about the existence and possible source of any problems.

Did I Divorce Him Too Soon?

After reading *Male Menopause,* I wondered if I had not been too quick in giving my husband a divorce. I asked for it after having found out he was having an affair. He was fifty-four and I was forty-six. I was going through the change myself and was not giving him much TLC. We didn't really talk much about what was happening. I was so hurt, I just wanted him out of my life. Two years ago, he died. I miss him very, very much and am hurt that I cannot talk to him about what happened to us.

Michelle

Points of understanding:

• When a woman finds out a man is having an affair, it is devastating. Her first response is to blame herself or to blame the man.

The first can lead to self-destructive depression, the latter to destroying the relationship. Every marriage is different. Understanding male menopause can help the woman and man decide how best to heal a serious breach of trust.

• Most couples don't have to deal with the death of a spouse shortly after a relationship ends. Yet, death is a possibility for any of us at any time. It's a good practice to live as if this is our last day and make decisions as if those they affect might not always be around.

Tragedy—A Grandfather Goes to Prison

Five years ago, our children came to our house in the middle of the night. They asked their father if he had abused two of our grandchildren. He did not deny it and turned himself in to the authorities. He received treatment for six months before he was incarcerated and was doing well.

The whole family was astonished to learn of my husband's behavior. Here is a man who raised six children, worked two jobs, was a good husband, and, at the age of fifty-seven, offended against two children aged eight and thirteen. No one could help us understand why this happened until we read your article.

In the years before the offense occurred, Joseph had lost his parents in a train accident, his brother-in-law to a massive heart attack, and his best friend was killed suddenly in a freak skiing accident. He never really confronted his feelings and our sex life was practically over. He was unhappy at work, but didn't feel he could quit or find something else at his age. He went to his doctor, who gave him an antidepressant, asked him if he was having an affair, dismissed his concerns, and sent him on his way. The doctor's attitude only increased his feelings of hopelessness.

Joseph has participated in the rehabilitation programs for five years, been a good role model at the correctional institution, and has done all he can to rectify his errors. Yet, every time he comes up for parole, his application is denied.

Every symptom that you had in your article fit Joseph for the last ten years except for the offending, which occurred six months before he was confronted. I only wish we had known sooner what was going on. Perhaps the outcome would have been different. However, all we can do is be supportive and love him until and after he comes home.

Dana

Points of understanding:

• Let me be clear at the outset that I am not blaming child abuse on male menopause. There are many reasons that men (and women) abuse children. None are justified and children must be protected. When we hear the term "child abuser" we often close our mind to the person behind the label.

• Symptoms of male menopause, if not understood and dealt with, can later have a variety of serious consequences. Men, even when they get the courage to go to the doctor, are often not taken seriously. They are told, "You're just getting older, what do you expect," or, "Take a Prozac and call me in the morning."

• All people who interact with men—wives, lovers, children, friends, doctors—need to listen more closely to what men are saying and to what they aren't saying. Often, men speak in silences, in "beady eyes," or limp penises. We need to listen closely to the truth that is beyond words.

• Male menopause, if not taken seriously, can cause tremendous grief and pain to a man and his family. Don't wait until a disaster occurs. Ask for help now to prevent further problems later.

Male Menopause Calls Out to a Couple in Their Twenties

I just finished reading *Male Menopause* and I must say, it was incredible!

I am a wife and mother, and although I am twenty-one and my husband is twenty-three, I felt this book calling my name.

I have loved my husband wholeheartedly, and earnestly longed to learn more about him. I particularly want to know about his health and what role I will play later in his life. As I have read this book, I have discussed what I've learned with my husband. Even though I didn't think it was possible, we have become so much closer.

We have agreed to welcome the "Menopause Passage," and embrace the fantastic changes of our lives.

And yes, you have helped someone understand that you can conquer "second adulthood" and survive.

Jane

Points of understanding:

• If everyone began to learn about the stages men go through when they were in their early twenties, think how many problems people would be able to avoid in their forties and fifties.

• Since we will all go through this time of life, it pays to be ready as soon as possible. It's like having a life insurance policy all paid up for when you need it.

Why Do Most Women Know More about Male Menopause Than Most Men?

Women are tuned into their own bodies early in life. They recognize that changes can occur from the inside as well as from outside forces. When a man is in a bad mood, he will more likely look to problems on the job or stresses with his family than shifts inside his own body. We all owe a debt of gratitude to women researchers who have taken the lead in helping us recognize the reality of male menopause.

It was in Rosetta Reitz's book *Menopause: A Positive Approach*, that I first read a sensitive account of male menopause. Reitz's book was one of the early books on menopause, published in 1977. In it she describes her interviews with women from twenty-five to ninety-five years of age who spoke out on sex and aging, lovemaking, hormones, nutrition, and male midlife changes.

Reitz points out that the term "menopause" applies to the ending of a woman's monthly menstrual cycles, but it is really much more than that. "Menopause has come to mean a combination of elements a woman experiences at the same time her menstrual flow stops."

"We can apply the term to men, too, even if they don't menstruate," says Reitz. "For it is more the combination of life's circumstances that occur around the age of fifty, sometimes beginning as early as forty for some, that creates the condition labeled menopause."

Most of the women I interviewed for my book said, "It's about time men finally figured out that they have hormonal changes, just like we do."

Why Are Men So Angry and Depressed at This Time of Life?

For men going through male menopause, anger is often a cover for their deep unhappiness and depression. Depression often covers over a great deal of rage men feel. Here's how one man described it: "I felt like my world was falling apart. I got sick more often and worried about becoming incapacitated. I worried constantly about losing my job, my family, my wife, my strength. I was sure I had to figure things out myself so I didn't talk to anyone. Everything irritated me. It felt like my wife was going out of her way to make my life miserable, even though she claimed she was just trying to help. Most of the time I felt like I was about to explode so I just tried to keep my feelings locked inside. I know it didn't work, that I would leak anger constantly, but I didn't know what to do about it. My wife often told me I seemed depressed and suggested I see a doctor. That made me even more angry. I knew I'd be better if she'd just be a more loving wife."

Although depression is very common during this stage, men often deny they are depressed. They think of depression as being sad and weepy, apathetic, or suicidal. For them, the problems seem to be caused by someone else. "Someone is doing it to me. Who wouldn't be pissed," he screams in his mind or at his wife.

This is a time of major upheaval for men and they are totally unprepared to deal with it. Many women report that it was as if a switch was thrown and the nice, stable man he used to be turned into an angry, ungrateful, demanding monster. Think back on your children when they moved from childhood into adolescence and you'll remember the power of these changes.

Male menopause is much more disruptive for most men because there is so much more life experience that needs to change and so little understanding about what this change of life is about. They need love, compassion, and most of all information about what it is they are going through.

He Has Never Hurt Me, But I Am Concerned

I visited your Internet site on the subject of male menopause. I am concerned about this issue because of the changes I have been seeing in my husband. He is forty-seven, soon to be forty-eight, and there have been some big changes in his/our lives. He quit smoking this past December, but long before that, his level of patience began to diminish noticeably. He has become very hard to live with. He becomes enraged so easily. It seems that he wants very little to do with me and when we try to spend time together, it is "empty."

All he seems to care about is his job, his computer language classes, and spending time on his computer—he plays games with our son or he spends time on the Internet.

Whenever there is something around the house that requires his attention, he seems to get angry at me for bringing it up. But if I do something that is generally his job, like fixing the sink, he suddenly becomes enraged.

It has become difficult for him to do many physical tasks that were once easy for him. I know he is in a lot of pain, though he doesn't talk about it. We are concerned that there is something wrong (arthritis or lupus), but he refuses to see a doctor.

But all that aside, his anger/rage has really caused a wide "distance" between us. He has never hurt me, yet, but that thought is in my mind nonetheless. The fear is eroding our relationship. I have told you all of these things to say this…my marriage is in great trouble and I don't know what to do. His personality changes are very noticeable. He isn't the same person and I don't understand what is going on! Can you please help?

Dorothy

Points of understanding:

• Irritability and anger are two of the most common early warning signs of male menopause. While a man can be irritable and angry throughout his life, now it seems that everything bothers him—what his wife wears, whether the children call too often or not enough, if he is asked to do things around the house, or if he is not asked.

• Underlying the irritability, anger, and rage is the fear that he is "losing it"—his physical abilities, mental capabilities, competitive edge, sexual prowess, or his general health. Men who had felt the most capable and productive often feel the most anger when their abilities begin to slip away.

• Anger at the spouse is his way of saying, "I'm afraid. I don't know what to do. I need you to help me, but I'm angry that I need your help. I hate that I'm going through this and that you see me falling apart. I just wish you'd go away and leave me to die." But he doesn't say any of this, he just gets angrier and creates distance.

• Understanding, patience, and gentle touching are the most important, and difficult, things you can offer at this time of life.

He Feels Like Giving Up

My husband is forty-four and for the past two years has been dealing with what has been diagnosed as depression.

This was a man involved in family, a strong work ethic, high energy, committed entirely to his children ages fifteen, thirteen, and eight. Two years ago, it was as if someone flipped a switch—he became anxious, had trouble sleeping, and felt more and more anxiety over his career.

The doctor prescribed antidepressants, but he had terrible side effects, and stopped taking them. My fear is that he will simply give up. I noticed your "Dear Abby" article and so much of it hit home as to his fears—losing his children, career, aging parents, etc.

The article gave us some hope, but I feel we are hanging over a cliff. Please, if you can help, this is most urgent. He is in another relapse state where he has cycled so low and is feeling on the verge of giving up, I just don't know what to do for him.

Roxanne

Points of understanding:

• Many people have the feeling that a switch is being flipped. One day he is OK, the next he has changed. Although male menopause is a dramatic change, there are many warning signs that often go unnoticed.

• Understanding what is going on with men is difficult because, as my colleague Warren Farrell says, "Women can't hear what men don't say." And many men don't really know what is going on inside them.

What Is Depression?

The *American Medical Association Encyclopedia of Medicine* defines depression as "feelings of sadness, hopelessness, pessimism, and a general loss of interest in life, combined with a sense of reduced emotional well-being."

Depressed people have often been told to "just cheer up." But we know now that isn't possible because depression is caused by a disruption in the chemistry of the brain. Only by restoring chemical balance can we truly hope to cure depression. We now know that there is a strong inborn component to depression and that the susceptibility to depression runs in families.

Over the years I have been a therapist, I have found a real difference between the way women and men experience depression. For women, the predominant feeling is *sadness*, but for men, the predominant feeling is often *anger*.

Women often express their depression by blaming themselves. Men often express their depression by blaming others—their wives, bosses, the economy, the government—anyone or anything but themselves. This was true in my own life. It wasn't until I recognized that my irritability, anger, and blame were manifestations of depression that I was finally able to ask for help and receive treatment.

He Assumed I'd Want a Divorce

I believe my husband is experiencing male menopause.

My husband attended a training away from home for five weeks (the end of August and beginning of September). He wanted me to visit during his third week, which I did. It was like a romantic getaway for both of us. I returned home regretfully, but had to get back to work. He returned two weeks later and things have not been the same since.

I knew there was something wrong when I met him at the airport. He was very moody, said nothing was wrong, and wouldn't talk. When we made love, he found it difficult to obtain an erection and asked me to be patient with him. I have really tried to do this, but I love him deeply and need to know what is happening.

I keep asking him what is wrong, but he just gets irritated and pulls away when I try to touch him. We have had sex a few times, I say sex because it is not lovemaking, it *must* be in the middle of the night, in the dark and he will nudge me and push at me to notice he has an erection, but will not reach out to me. The sex has become abusive, the last time he made me feel like a prostitute.

Many things have happened in the past two years. He retired from the U.S. Army. He went to work for a large corporation that works with the government on defense contracts. We bought our first home (it is out in the country and quite a drive for both of us, but we agreed it would be worth it). And our only child (a daughter) got married two weeks ago.

Yesterday, I finally got him to talk to me about what is troubling him. He said that the week before he was to return home, he realized he didn't want to come home, that he was unhappy with his work and his life. He said he still loves me but wants to be on his own working as a contractor traveling for a while.

He had already made all these plans and decided for me that I would automatically want a divorce. I told him that we should have been talking about this from the beginning, and he said that now he realized that he should have been more open and he should have been talking to me. He told me that he is being selfish, immature, knows he is hurting me and our family, but that he still wants to go away.

He also said that he loves me and wants to stay married to me, that he would like for me to take him back when he returns. He admits that he has been purposely pushing me away emotionally so that it will be easier on me when he leaves. I love this man with all my heart, I am so hurt and I do not know what to do. I would like to go with him and always be with him, but he doesn't want that at this time. (He really loved being in the Army and traveling. We traveled extensively while he was in the Army and lived many places.) My husband, daughter, and I have always been very close. Before his training trip, my husband and I had been talking about the two of us eventually traveling overseas to work again and suddenly he doesn't want me along.

I am very confused, very hurt, very everything. I cannot sleep or eat. I cry a lot. I can't do my work for worry. I know he is feeling exactly the same, but he won't admit it. He said he will work it out. He is worth fighting for, but I do not know how to do it. Please help me.

Jill

Points of understanding

• When a man is depressed and confused, he often expresses it with anger and irritation.

• The more a woman asks what's wrong, the more a man feels increasing pressure and withdraws. He often doesn't know what's wrong and feels guilty because he is irritated, and guilty because he doesn't understand what's going on.

• Sex, at these times, is used more as a release of tension than as a way to connect emotionally and lovingly.

• Male menopause is often precipitated by major life changes that seem to be "good," but are often very stressful.

• Many men feel a need to escape from their old life, but feel ashamed of the desire and so don't talk about it.

• They often need a way to go off on their own, to find the meaning for the second half of their lives. In Native American cultures, it was called a Vision Quest. We need to find ways of reinstituting this form of life transition for adolescent boys and midlife men.

How Serious Is Depression and Do Men and Women Experience It Differently?

I believe too many men, particularly in the midlife years, are suffering and dying from unrecognized depression. I find the following facts disturbing:

• 80 percent of all suicides in the United States are men.

• The rate of suicide for men forty-five to sixty-four is three times higher than the rate for women of the same age. For men over sixty-five, the rate is nearly seven times higher.

• A large Swedish survey found a history of depression multiplied the risk for suicide seventy-eight fold compared to those with no such history.

• If you're forty-five, in perfect health, and depressed, you're somewhere between 50 percent and 100 percent more likely to have a heart attack than if you weren't depressed. And if you have a heart attack and then get depressed, whether you simply get some symptoms of depression or the full diagnosis, over the next eighteen months, you are three and one-half times more likely to die.

• There are roughly five hundred thousand heart attacks a year in the U.S., and 20 percent of the heart attack victims develop depression.

• Mood disorders are the "common cold" of mind/body illnesses and more than twenty million Americans will suffer an episode of depression during their lifetimes.

• Since the turn of the century, each successive generation has doubled its susceptibility to depression.

• Sixty to 80 percent of people with depression never get help.

• Men often think of depression as a "woman's ailment" and are reluctant to seek help even when they know they are suffering.

• Most men are not aware that they are depressed and so never have the opportunity to get help.

• Depressed men, particularly those over fifty, rarely voice any intent to commit suicide before they actually try to kill themselves. They die silently with no one even knowing how hopeless they were feeling.

Why Are Men Prone to Mood Swings at This Stage?

Men going through male menopause can go from being the nicest, gentlest guys to acting like monsters in the bat of an eye. It's like they were raw nerves. When they're touched one way, they respond in a loving manner. When they're touched another way, they respond with anger. Often they don't respond at all. If that weren't bad enough, it's never clear what's going to bring out the joy and what's going to bring out the irritation. Something that made them happy one day is irritating the next.

For those around them, they need to be patient, have their own lives on a steady course so they don't go up and down like a roller coaster, and be patient beyond belief. It often helps to have counseling.

One Minute He Loves Us, the Next He Wants to Leave

I am thirty-nine, and my boyfriend is forty-one years old. I have a twenty-year-old daughter who is living with us.

He and I met three years ago and hit it off immediately. We had lots in common. We loved to walk and hike, camp and kayak, anything outdoors. He moved in with us and things were wonderful until about a year ago when he started getting mad at me for every little thing I said or did. Though I practically worship him, he would say I don't love and respect him.

When we'd get into fights he'd tell me to leave, but when I'd start packing he'd say he didn't mean it. Things would be wonderful for awhile. He seemed like the same loving guy I first met, then it was like a dark bank of clouds would roll in and his moods would shift. It was like Jekyll and Hyde. I never knew if he was going to be a loving man or an angry monster.

He has a bad back and in the past would ask me to massage it for him, which I loved to do. Now he accuses me of not caring about his back, but when I offer to rub him, he yells, "I took care of myself fine all these years before I met you, I can take care of myself now." Lately, he spends more time doing things without me, telling me he just needs some space for himself.

When I started doing things without him for the sole purpose of letting him have his own space, he told me I was ignoring him, that I never had time for him anymore. When I pointed out that I was just giving him the space he was asking for, he flew into a rage and accused me of being with other men, which is totally ridiculous. He began following me and finally "caught me" on a beach where I had been kayaking with my daughter. After that he's been especially nice to us both. I think he feels guilty and confused, but neither of us knows what's going on. Help! Is this male menopause? My men friends at work think it is.

Gena

Points of understanding:

• When men are going through male menopause they are very vulnerable and often feel a lack of love and respect even when it is freely given.

• There is often an approach-avoidance dance, where he wants you to leave one minute and begs you to stay the next. He pushes you away with one hand and pulls you close with the other. Like an adolescent, he both wants his freedom and is terrified to be on his own.

• He feels vulnerable to physical changes and feels he's "falling apart" if he has any ailments. Asking for help is like an admission of weakness and failure. He wants and needs your support, but has difficulty accepting it.

• He can be extremely jealous and fearful. His own fantasies of freedom are often projected on his partner and he accuses her of doing what "he wants" to do. However, the proverbial search for a young, beautiful female is not simply a desire for sex. It often has more to do with finding something to take away his pain. It also is an attempt to break from his old life-patterns and find a new direction for his life.

He Is Acting Completely Out of Character

Help! I thought we had one of the best marriages around until two months ago. My husband just turned fifty and we have gone through a lot in the past five years: rape of a daughter and her resulting eating disorder and pregnancy, terrible financial hardship, depression, and a debilitating on-the-job injury.

Finally, after being off work a long time, my husband is being retrained. He has been in the house a lot for the past two years and even though he was depressed and hurt, I was his everything. I supported, nurtured and comforted him whenever he needed it. We would go out together every weekend and really enjoy each other's company.

In the last two months when he started school, I noticed a change. I would ask him about it and he would say it was nothing until finally he broke down and told me he was losing feelings for me. That was shocking as we had been so close and always there for each other despite all the many pressures we have had in life.

Now he has an attitude with me and does not want to answer to me or be accountable. I can see that he truly still loves me, although he verbally is saying something different.

He told me the other night that he is going to save money and move out, but there is no other woman. He says he wants to move back to San Diego, where we are from, but isn't sure if he wants to move back together, though he assures me he doesn't want a divorce. I realize he has been through a lot, but why the sudden turn on his best friend, the one who has always been there for him? I am confused and very upset. He is acting completely out of character.

Karen

Points of understanding:

• For men, work can become such a large part of our identity, when we are out of work we feel like our very existence is threatened.

• Depression is very common for men at this age as losses of various kinds take their toll.

• Whenever I hear a woman say or suggest that, "I was his everything," I know there is going to be trouble. When a man leans too heavily on a woman, he eventually will resent her and seek freedom to show he can still stand on his own feet.

• Many women say that the men in their lives are "acting completely out of character." Male menopause is a time of transition from first adulthood to second adulthood. We wouldn't expect an adolescent boy to act in the same character as a ten-year-old. The male menopause transition is every bit as powerful as adolescence. Prepare for men to "act out" in some way. Male menopause is as natural and as difficult as going through puberty.

He Said He Had Nowhere to Go

My husband is forty-six years old and we have been married for twenty years. Shortly before our anniversary this past August, I noticed he seemed distant and somewhat irritable, and for him, almost nasty. Our marriage before this has been rather ordinary. I thought the reason for his mood was due to stress, mostly financial, but I assumed things would be OK.

When I finally approached him about it, he simply said he didn't feel anything anymore and would really like to be on his own. He said he felt like he missed out on that as a younger guy, but that his age now doesn't bother him. He says he's fine with it. He keeps saying he wants to come and go as he pleases which he has never done before.

After awhile I also found he was developing a "relationship" with someone sixteen years younger than him. When we had a blowup over it, he broke it off completely. Then I found out he had already had a consultation with a lawyer. But he didn't take any concrete steps towards leaving.

In anger, I attempted to throw him out, but he said he had nowhere to go. He seems very confused and at times prefers to get lost in work. I left your article for him and he took it with him, and did ask me for other articles I had gathered on saving marriages.

He is friendly most of the time, but refuses to be touched and seems to have distanced himself from our nineteen-year-old son.

He seems so different from the man I've loved for so long. I guess what I need to know is how do I get him to get help and where do we go? I am desperate, as I love him dearly and see his pain as much as the pain he is causing this family.

Laura

Points of understanding:

• Men often feel they missed out on many things during the time they worked hard to be good family men. Their frustration, anger, disappointment, guilt, and shame are often not expressed. Burying these feelings may cause him to become numb and disconnected.

• Getting involved with a younger woman is often the only way a man knows to reconnect with his feelings. He doesn't want to end a marriage, but rather to break through the frozen river of feelings and get them flowing again.

• He's caught between a rock and a hard place. He knows he needs to make a major change in his life, but he doesn't want to leave the marriage. His life hangs in the balance until he can get the kind of support that will make sense to him.

• These changes affect the whole family. Men fear that their wives and children would disapprove and abandon them if they ever voiced their desire to remake their lives.

• Recognizing his pain, as well as the pain he is causing others, is the first step to getting the help a family needs.

Why Do Men Want to Leave Their Wives or Have Affairs at This Time of Life?

All men and women are different and there is no single answer that will be true for everyone. However, there seems to be a common theme I hear in men going through male menopause. In various ways, they are saying, "I want to be free, I want to be me." Like teenagers who need to fight their way out of the world of childhood in order to take their place in the world, men need to let go of the old world of first adulthood in order to take their place as maturing adults in the second half of life.

Like teenagers who often rebel against their parents, men often rebel against their families. They see their wives and children (even adult children) as trying to keep them chained to the past. They fantasize ways of escaping, not realizing that the real change must occur inside, not by running away. Getting a divorce or finding a younger woman gets their juices flowing and gives them the illusion that everything is OK.

They usually find out that they still have to deal with male menopause, but without help, they often withdraw and shut down inside.

He Is Not Acting Like Himself

Is Bill Clinton's involvement with Monica Lewinsky related to his "midlife" crisis? And why would he choose Monica? Is she reflecting to him his "unresolved" adolescent issues?

I thought perhaps you could give some insight on this. My husband, fifty-one, has decided he needed to leave a twenty-seven-year relationship with me after obsessing for a year or so about a younger woman who was pursuing him…and he sounds and acts totally "unlike himself."

Actually, this younger woman is totally unsuited to my husband—she is very needy, which I am not—sort of like Monica isn't suited to the "leader of the free world." Now, if Bill Clinton had picked Sharon Stone or someone similar, it would be more understandable to me.

My husband just sort of walked away from a "very good and close" family life in order to "date" this younger, needy woman who pursued him in various ways for over a year. He and I enjoyed a good sex life, but over the past year he was basically isolating me and thinking about the other woman. He lost interest in his hobbies, was not present in spirit, and basically seemed depressed but refused to accept his feelings and actions.

He also became a pathological liar during that time. In other words, a high-class guy was acting in low-class ways. His behavior was characterized by extreme mood swings and impulsive actions. I hope you have some insight.

Andrea

Points of understanding:

• Many women are absolutely amazed at the kind of women that men are attracted to at midlife. The media image is that men are attracted to a Playboy bunny to ride in his red Corvette and fulfill all his sexual fantasies. The reality is that most men who look elsewhere at this time of life are looking for a woman who will listen to their pain and heartache, offer a new opportunity for life, need him, and make him feel important.

• Men, who have often been the ones who pursued women throughout their lives, love the feeling of being pursued. If she is young and pretty and reminds him of the kind of woman he was not able to attract in his younger days, he easily can become obsessed.

• As we know, from the Joe next door to the president of the United States, men can make fools of themselves when they are in the thrall of hormonal changes, whether they occur in adolescence or midlife. The good news is that if men and women can understand male menopause, much of the insanity can be avoided and lived through.

I'm Living a Nightmare

I'm living a nightmare. I want to save my marriage, but I don't know what to do. He says he just doesn't love us and wants out. He got involved with a younger woman four years ago and I haven't known what to do. We tried marriage counseling, but that didn't seem to help.

We've been together for twenty-eight years, but now it looks like the marriage is falling apart. What's even worse is I don't know why it's happening.

He began having sexual problems two years ago, but we've been having communication problems for a long time. We were both workaholics, trying to build up our business. We really had no personal life. Everything was put into expanding and growing the business.

For many years, it was wonderful working together. We were partners on an adventure and even when we were away from each other, we felt connected. But over the years, we began to grow apart. As he moved away, I became more involved in my own work. When he asked me once if I still loved him, I was honest and said, "I love you, but I'm not 'in love' with you." I knew it hurt him, but it was the truth. I just felt numb inside. I wanted to get through to him, to let him know how much I missed him and how I wanted us to regain the love and passion we once had.

On one of the trips overseas he was rumored to have gotten involved with a young woman who worked in the local office. When he returned, he told me he was considering moving there to live.

I couldn't believe what I was hearing. You must be crazy, I thought. This can't be happening. I thought we had an ideal marriage and a great family. Now it seemed like he didn't like us anymore and just wanted to get away.

Della

Points of understanding:

• In the early years of marriage, men and women are often so focused on work and family that they neglect nurturing the relationship.

• Sexual behavior outside the marriage is usually preceded by sexual problems inside the marriage. Problems inside marriage are usually preceded by a loss of communication and intimacy between the couple.

• Men are often much more vulnerable than they let on. Telling him "I love you, but am not in love with you" may feel more like a devastating rejection than an invitation to heal a relationship that has grown apart.

• Women, like men, often neglect to notice or deny the deep unhappiness men feel and then are surprised when their "ideal" marriage falls apart.

Things Just Seem So Dead

I'm fifty-three and my wife is forty-eight. We've been having difficulties for the last three or four years. I'll tell you, I believe in being honest. I'm not going to make excuses for what happened. In spite of the difficulties between us, I believe I have been moral and true to my wife, Della. I haven't had sex with any other woman, though I have been tempted. It's true I was thinking of getting a divorce and moving away. I entertained dreams of living abroad.

I know this may sound strange, but I had reached a saturation point. We had built a worldwide business and had offices in many countries. Two of our three sons and our daughter work in the business, and it's something we wanted to leave as a legacy to the kids. But I've gotten to where I just don't care anymore.

I don't feel the same things I felt for Della. If you can help me recapture the lost feelings, I want to stay. I don't want to throw away my family. I have a fear that once I do, I'll miss what I have and want it back. But things just seem so dead. I need help.

Della went from being so supportive, the perfect mate and business partner, to this woman I don't even know. She's always critical now. I feel like she opposes me in everything. She's always nagging and I don't feel like I can do anything right.

In the past, we would often travel together, and when we didn't our partings and returnings were often the best part of the trips. Now there is tension when I leave and tension when I return.

One year ago, she said, "I'm not in love with you any more." When she said that, something died in me. Later, when I met the woman in Australia, she seemed to have all the qualities I wanted in a woman. Although I had taken vows with Della that I wasn't going to break, I felt so drawn to the other woman. She really seemed to like me just the way I was. It was so nice to be with someone who was comfortable to be with and who cared.

But I came back. I could see that it was really dishonorable the way I left and I told Della I wanted to see if we could work things out. Now, it seems she has made a 180 degree turn and is being totally supportive and loving. I don't know if she's doing that because she really feels it, or just to keep me close. It's very confusing.

Points of understanding:

• Most men have no idea that many of the difficulties they are having in their relationships are tied to male menopause.

• When they begin feeling the urge to break out of their old mold, they are often not aware of the nightmare it may cause in their families.

• Many men feel that if they are not actually having sex with another woman, but only thinking about it, or they haven't left their wives but only thought about getting a divorce and moving out, they are still being true to their relationship. Most men are genuinely confused. They feel caught between the old life that no longer works for them and a new life that hasn't yet been engaged.

• Many men find that the life they have built, the one that was supposed to take them through retirement and into the golden years is no longer satisfying, even if it is highly successful by outside standards. Not knowing how to make significant changes, they often feel the only choice is to escape.

• Emotions often become deadened as men push down feelings of anger, hurt, fear, guilt, shame, and despair. The result is that feelings of love and affection also may be cut off.

• Men often long for the feelings they felt in the past, long for a relationship that they had when they were young. When he doesn't feel it with his long-term partner, he often feels like something has died. He may blame her for the loss.

• At this stage of life, men are very sensitive and vulnerable. They feel criticized and unappreciated. This is often caused by a man not feeling good inside and being hypersensitive to words and deeds from his wife. It is also caused by wives who are becoming more assertive and less willing to keep their own feelings inside. The result may be a man who feels uncared for.

• Many men seek younger women, less for the sexual desire and more for the feelings that they are appreciated and loved just the way they are.

• Self-acceptance and acceptance of our spouse are two of the most difficult tasks of male menopause.

Is Male Menopause Just an Excuse for Men to Act Out?

Before I began research for my book, I had heard a number of people talk about male menopause, but wondered if they were just complaining about the difficulties of being a man or trying to justify their irresponsible midlife behavior. In a society where more and more people see themselves as victims, it wouldn't surprise me for some people to look for an excuse for their behavior.

As a therapist, I have little tolerance for men (or women) who bemoan their lives or who blame bad behavior on something or someone other than themselves.

However, after studying male menopause, I know now it is as real as what women experience as their hormone levels change. Although we all need to be held accountable for our actions, men's behavior during this time needs to be understood, not judged. Often, "acting out" is the only way a man knows to break out of his past patterns. With greater understanding, he may find better ways of making this vital life transition.

How Should Men in This Stage of Life Deal with Their Medical Concerns?

Men need to be willing to be real advocates for their own health, to seek out the best supports available. If one approach doesn't satisfy, they need to try others. Don't be afraid to ask questions.

I've Had Good Health and Vitality Until This Illness

After reading your article, I realize I've had this problem for years. I am finally being treated by an endocrinologist, but she is puzzled. I am using an androderm 5 mg patch. It minimized my problems but did not cure them. I had most of the symptoms you indicated: indecisiveness; weight gain; short-term memory loss; sleep disturbances; reduced libido; flushness of the neck, face, and scalp; and tired feelings. My testosterone level is in the low range still, even after using the testosterone patch.

I am a seventy-three-year-old veteran and have been fortunate to have had good health and vitality until this illness.

Sanford

Points of understanding:

• Unlike women who often have a gynecologist to address menopausal needs, there is no comparable specialist for men. My friend James Green, only half jokingly, suggests that we need a "guy-necologist" to help men with their special needs. At present, some men see their general practitioner or internist, others go to a urologist, while some make their way to an endocrinologist. What makes things even more complicated is that male menopause is not primarily a medical problem. I believe there are hormonal, physical, psychological, interpersonal, social, sexual, and spiritual dimensions that are all equally important and each aspect needs to be addressed for total understanding.

• With male menopause just becoming understood, many men only recognize it when they've had it a long time. As we learn more, hopefully men will seek support much sooner.

Male Menopause in Full Swing

After reading your article, I have concluded that my male menopause is in full swing at age fifty-six. In addition to the symptoms you mention, the following are of major concern to me and my wife.

• The prostate surgery I had more than a year ago.

• The hernia operation six months later kept me in bed longer than it should have.

• My erectile dysfunction is getting worse.

• I have a prescription for Viagra, but I haven't used it.
• This has caused frustration for both my wife and myself.
• I am working full-time, but am enjoying it less and less.
• My energy level feels too low.
• My wife and I have gone several years without sex.

Any suggestions would be helpful.

Felix

Points of understanding:

• Felix is like a lot of men who contact me. They're not much interested in what caused the problem, how they feel about it, or seeing the larger picture of what the symptoms mean in their lives. It's like taking their car into the repair shop. "Here's what's wrong, fix it, send me the bill." Fortunately, or unfortunately, the human body is so much more complex than a car. We need to understand the way all the parts work together.

• Prostate surgery is a significant event. What was the cause—benign enlargement, cancer? What lead up to the problem? What kind of surgery was it? How successful was it? How did he cope? These are a few questions doctors should ask.

• A hernia surgery coming six months later can add to the stress. What caused the surgery? How long did it take to heal? How long "should" it have taken? Men often feel that their bodies should heal like twenty-year-olds when we are in our fifties.

• How long has the erectile dysfunction been going on? What's the nature of the dysfunction—not able to get an erection, keep it long enough for sexual enjoyment, losing it too soon, ejaculating too late or too early? There's so much that needs to be known about a complex subject like a man's ejaculation. It's not like fixing the fuel injection system in his sedan.

• Why has he not used his Viagra prescription? Is he afraid it won't work, that it will put more pressure on him and the relationship? Viagra can be helpful, but it isn't magic. Doctors need to understand so much about a man and his relationship to see what would be most helpful.

• Frustration often builds up when the full picture of what is going on with a man is not clear. It's like the proverbial blind men trying to understand what they're dealing with by touching different parts of an elephant. If we don't look at the whole man, we are sure to become frustrated.

• Work is often the cornerstone of a man's earlier life. When that begins to change as he gets older, it can be confusing. Losing interest in one's work can either be seen as a downward slide to loss of interest in life, or it can be an indication that a man needs to move on to what I call his "soul's calling."

• Like the trapeze artist who must let go of the bar they are holding before they can "fly" to the next bar, a man often has to let go of the old job before he can find what is calling him in the second half of life. Even if he knows what that new calling might be, which most of us don't know initially, letting go can be frightening.

• Low energy is one of the defining signs of male menopause. It is a signal that the old ways are not working and there is a need to slow down, and look inward.

• Sexual difficulties have many causes, such as hormonal shifts, physical illnesses, medications, depression, relationship problems, and low self-esteem. They also can be an indication that it is time to move from "first adulthood sexuality" to "second adulthood sexuality." In first adulthood, sexuality is often focused on "procreation." At this stage, men are designed to want to have sex frequently with hard erections that last a long time and return frequently. In second adulthood, sexuality is more focused on "co-creation." At this stage, we are more interested in intimacy, sensuality, and playfulness.

• Couples who are not being sexual, and this is true of a surprising number of couples, need to understand what this means in their lives. This is a difficult area for most men and women to discuss. Having a counselor trained in these issues may be helpful.

Attention Deficit and Hyperactivity Disorder and Male Menopause

My husband is experiencing some of the symptoms of male menopause including hot flashes and periods of perspiring that he doesn't understand. He recently read your book and recognized himself throughout. He is fifty-three years old and I am fifty-one. I'm also going through menopause which makes it doubly difficult.

He was diagnosed with attention deficit and hyperactivity disorder (ADHD) with impulsivity in October 1996. We have been in counseling to help us understand ADHD and its effects on our relationship. We have been married thirty years. I love him with all my heart and it hurts seeing him feeling so badly about himself. He grew up in a family that did not understand him. He did not have a very good relationship with either of his parents but his relationship with his mother was especially difficult. She had ADHD also.

Since about age forty, he has suffered with some depression and also feels he is not the "man he used to be." Physically, he isn't quite like he was in his twenties, but to me he is fantastic. It doesn't matter how I feel about him though—it's how he feels about himself that counts and I can't change that.

Dealing with life changes the past ten years is another challenge for him. He would like to see a doctor that understands male menopause. He went to a doctor in our area, but his doctor said he knew nothing about the subject. The doctor said he wasn't sure it existed. My husband has lost confidence in the medical profession in regard to his problems and is embarrassed to see anyone else for help. Thank you for listening.

Joy

Points of understanding:

• ADD or ADHD was once thought to effect mostly boys. They couldn't seem to sit still in school, were impulsive, aggressive, and inattentive. There was, and still is, a great deal of controversy about whether these boys needed medications like Ritalin or were just being boys in a school system that didn't attend to their needs.

• Now we recognize that ADD or ADHD are the tip of a large clinical "iceberg" that often does not disappear in childhood, but continues into adulthood, and effects females as well as males. It is increasingly clear that there is a neurochemical basis for these disorders.

• The most prominent feature of all these disorders is emotional and physical hypersensitivity. These people often are sensitive to various forms of "chaos" and react with hyperactivity, rages, addictive behaviors, compulsive sexual acting out, excessive worry, and depression in their unsuccessful attempts to cope.

• Though some people have these problems throughout their lives, others find that the changes brought about by male menopause can trigger many of these reactions. There is often a need to understand and treat these problems together if a man is to successfully complete the male menopause passage.

• Many doctors don't understand male menopause or ADHD in adults. I've listed a number of resources at the back of this book that will help you in finding the help you need.

What Do Changes in Testosterone Levels Have to Do with Male Menopause?

It's been called the "hormone from hell" and "the fountain of youth." It is blamed for wars, gang violence, rape, and the body and mind of Sylvester Stallone. It is credited with making men strong, shrinking their bellies, protecting their heart, and boosting sexual desire in both men and women. It is perhaps the most misunderstood player in the human sexual symphony. It is what makes those born with an XY chromosome, male. It is testosterone. Here's how it works.

In the first weeks in the womb, the tiny fetus is neither male nor female. It has all the basic equipment to develop as either sex. At around six weeks, the sexual identity is finally determined and, if it is male, the special cells in the testes produce male hormones, the main one being testosterone. It helps craft the penis, the scrotum, and testicles, along with the contouring of the body—very valuable additions if you are a male.

We don't get much action from this hormone until it is awakened with a bang when the boy reaches puberty and testosterone levels rise 400 to 1000 percent. "Teenage boys become walking grenades, just waiting to go off," says Theresa Crenshaw, M.D., author of *The Alchemy of Love and Lust*, and an expert on hormonal changes in men and women. "As production kicks into high gear, the psychological and physical impact of testosterone is overwhelming. More than any other substance, testosterone controls the development and maintenance of masculine characteristics."

Many people blame testosterone for the aggression and violence that we see in men. This blame, I believe, is unfounded. The problem is not testosterone, but rather our societal inability to guide and direct the energy of young males, with their surging testosterone, into constructive channels.

As men age, their testosterone levels fall. This is one of the chief markers of male menopause and it contributes to the many symptoms we see in aging men, including loss of muscle mass and bone density.

Do Men Experience Hormonal Cycles?

Lowered levels of hormones at midlife are central to the changes associated with male menopause. Testosterone is one of the significant hormones that decreases as men age, but there are testosterone cycles that occur throughout a man's life.

We now know that men, like women, experience complex hormonal rhythms that affect their sexuality, mood, and temperament. For instance, researchers have found five different testosterone cycles in men:

• Rhythmic fluctuations three to four times an hour. (Could this account for research that shows that men think about sex every fifteen minutes?)

• Daily changes with testosterone higher in the morning and lower in the afternoon.

• Fluctuations throughout the year with levels higher in October and lower in April.

• Decreasing levels associated with male menopause that occur as men get older.

• Monthly fluctuations that are rhythmic.

"The morning highs, daily fluctuations, and seasonal cycles whip men around," says Dr. Crenshaw. "Think about the moment-to-moment impact of testosterone levels firing and spiking all over the place during the day, and what this must be doing to a man's temperament."

If Men Have Monthly Hormonal Cycles, Do They Get PMS?

Men, like women, have what could be called "PMS." They, too, have physical and emotional reactions to hormonal fluctuations throughout the month.

In a recent study, when men were given the same checklists of symptoms from a typical PMS questionnaire—omitting the female specific symptoms, such as breast tenderness—men reported having as many symptoms (reduced or increased energy, irritability, and other negative moods, back pain, sleeplessness, headaches, confusion, etc.) as women do—when the symptoms aren't called PMS.

Since writing *Male Menopause*, I have talked with a number of men who substantiate these findings. They are aware, though they have been reluctant to admit it, that their moods change depending on the time of month. One man said he has been keeping track of his "monthlies" for over a year and recognizes changes in mood, sexuality, and physical comfort at a particular time each month.

Is Taking Natural Testosterone a Way to Keep Men's Potency and Vitality Strong?

Some people believe that declining levels of testosterone are natural and need to be accepted. Others believe that replacing lost testosterone can restore men's vitality and virility. As with hormone replacement for women, this is a controversial area of research.

It's my belief that testosterone replacement therapy will become as prevalent as replacement of estrogen and progesterone has become for women. Although there are risks in taking testosterone when levels are low, there are also benefits.

Although there had long been treatments for ED, the advent of Viagra made treatment much easier. Taking a pill a half hour before making love was much easier, more comfortable, and "sexier" than getting a shot or using other intrusive means.

Likewise, there have been new discoveries in the area of testosterone research. For the first time, millions of testosterone-deficient men may have an alternative that will offer many of the benefits of testosterone replacement therapy that, like Viagra, is more comfortable than previous methods.

Unimed Pharmaceuticals now offers a product called AndroGel that shows great promise in helping menopausal men.

AndroGel is a clear, odorless topical gel proposed for once daily application to the upper arms and/or abdomen. It does not transfer from its application site, making it easy to wear clothing and be active without fear of the gel rubbing off.

This way of administering testosterone could prove as important for men with testosterone deficiency as Viagra has proved a help to men experiencing erectile dysfunction. Viagra helps with erections, but has no effect on sexual desire. Testosterone has many health benefits, including increased sexual desire. Both may prove to be a potent combination for helping men move through male menopause.

How Common Is Erectile Dysfunction for Men Going through Male Menopause?

Erectile dysfunction (ED) is defined as the persistent inability to attain and maintain an erection adequate to permit satisfactory sexual performance.

According to results from the Massachusetts Male Aging Study, who followed a large sample of men between the ages of forty and seventy, the combined prevalence of minimal, moderate, and complete erectile dysfunction was 52 percent.

Although the study found that psychological factors play a role, physical factors are more significant. There was a high correlation between ED and heart disease, hypertension, and diabetes, as well as with the medications that are often taken to deal with these problems.

Since the physical, psychological, and sexual aspects are interconnected, most of these symptoms can be prevented and treated by concentrating on the whole man.

Sex and Depression: How Can I Help Him?

My husband has recently been diagnosed with severe depression and has been told that he is going through male menopause. He is taking Celexa for the depression but if things weren't already bad enough, he is going through sexual difficulties now also. He can get an erection but he can't ejaculate. He is really down about this and I don't know what to do to help him. I am desperate. I am trying to save my marriage and my family. Please let me know what to do next or what I can try.

Lanie

Points of understanding:

• Sexual difficulties and depression often are a major part of male menopause and often are related. When we feel depressed, we have problems with sex and when we are having problems with sex we become depressed.

• Many medications, including antidepressants, may cause or increase problems with sexual functioning.

• A man and woman need to be patient with themselves and each other. They need to find a doctor who can work with them on medications and their effects and side effects. Good counseling should always be a part of a total health offering.

What Erection Changes Are Normal As Men Age?

If a man and his partner are not aware of the normal changes, they may become fearful that these changes are early signs of ED, begin worrying about it, and contribute to the very problems they want to prevent. Normal changes include:

• Erections take longer to occur.

• A man more often requires direct physical stimulation to get an erection, a sexy sight or fantasy may not arouse him as it once did.

• The full erection doesn't get quite as firm as when he was younger.

• His urge to ejaculate is not as insistent as before. Sometimes he doesn't feel like ejaculating at all.

• The force of ejaculation is not as strong as it was in the past. The amount of his ejaculate is less, and he may have fewer sperm.

Viagra: What Is It and What Can It Do to Help Men?

Viagra is a small blue pill that is used to treat ED. It is effective in treating erectile dysfunction caused by organic problems (such as diabetes or prostate cancer), psychological problems, or mixtures of organic and psychological problems.

It does not work for every man, nor is everyone a candidate to try it. The success rate varies from 60 percent to 80 percent depending on what is causing ED.

In clinical studies, Viagra was shown to be effective in helping men improve their sexual lives, specifically to help them achieve and maintain an erection sufficient for satisfactory sexual activity.

For most patients, the recommended dose is 50 mg taken as needed approximately one hour before sexual activity. However, Viagra may be taken anywhere from four hours to thirty minutes before sexual activity. Based on effectiveness and toleration, the dose may be increased to a maximum recommended dose of 100 mg or decreased to 25 mg. The maximum recommended dosing frequency is once per day.

Viagra works by prolonging the effects of a chemical, cGMP (by blocking an enzyme that breaks it down), which allows the smooth muscles in the spongy erectile tissues of the penis to relax, causing blood to enter the penis and produce an erection.

In clinical trials, the effects lasted up to four hours, but individual variation is great. A number of clients at our clinic say that they become easily aroused a second time within an hour after ejaculating.

Viagra: What Are the Dangers?

Though side effects were few, the following were reported along with the percentage experiencing the problem:

Headaches (16 percent)

Flushing (10 percent)

Digestive problems (7 percent)

Nasal Congestion (4 percent)

Urinary tract infection (3 percent)

Abnormal vision (3 percent)

Diarrhea (3 percent)

Dizziness (2 percent)

Rash (2 percent)

Viagra should not be taken by anyone who is also taking nitrate-based medications such as nitroglycerin. It should always be taken under the supervision of a competent medical doctor.

The main warning I offer is that if you do decide to take Viagra, or any other medication for treating erectile dysfunction, take it only under the supervision of a competent doctor who will give you a complete physical examination before prescribing the drug. Some doctors write prescriptions because patients demand the drug without taking proper precautions.

Among men seeking treatment for erectile dysfunction, physicians are now finding those who are also at high risk for heart disease. Finding these men early, even before they have had symptoms of heart disease, such as chest pain, gives doctors the opportunity to start them on therapies and counsel them on lifestyle changes aimed at preventing heart attack or sudden death due to heart disease.

Never buy Viagra online or use it without seeing your doctor first. Forty percent of men in one study seeking Viagra prescriptions were found to have significant coronary artery blockages.

We all would like to find quick solutions to long-time problems. But no one would want to get his erection back, only to lose his life because of an undiagnosed heart problem.

Why Is the Prostate Gland So Important for Men?

We can't talk about male menopause without talking about the penis and the prostate. The prostate is at the center of important systems in the male body—the urinary system and the sexual system.

The gland is about the size of a walnut and sits beneath the bladder. The urethra, which carries the urine from the bladder to the outside world for elimination, passes through the prostate.

First and foremost, the prostate is a sexual organ. It secretes and stores the fluid that makes up about one-third of the semen. This stored fluid is expressed out of the prostate at orgasm by muscular contractions of the gland and mixes with sperm and seminal fluid that allows for new life to form when sperm and egg connect. A healthy prostate is vital for having a joyful sexual experience.

We now know that the prostate gland is the most frequently diseased organ of the human body. All men are susceptible to contracting the three major diseases of the prostate:

1) Prostatitis (infection of the prostate)

2) Benign prostatic hyperplasia (BPH), also called enlarged prostate

3) Prostate cancer

As men move into male menopause, they are particularly concerned about BPH and prostate cancer.

Prostatitis, Hernias, and Erections

I was married for twenty-three years and during that time I had prostate problems and had my prostate trimmed at one time. I took medicine on a regular basis for prostatitis while I was married, and when I got divorced about eight years ago, the prostatitis went away. All doctors told me that my wife had nothing to do with my prostatitis although she had a lot of female problems.

My problem now is I'm having problems maintaining an erection in the mornings. I have tried Yohimbine which did not work. I tried Viagra and it didn't have any more effect than taking an aspirin.

Since I had a hernia operation about eighteen months ago, the erection problem has gotten worse. Can you help?

Bertram

Points of understanding:

• Prostatitis is a general term used for conditions that result in inflammation of the prostate gland. Usual symptoms include painful or burning urination and the need to void frequently. Although it is often treated as a purely physical ailment, symptoms can occur as a result of stress, marital, and sexual problems.

• Hernias and other physical illnesses and injury can have an effect on a man's erections.

• We often think of erections in men as happening automatically. Particularly in young men, it seemed that erections could be caused by anything and nothing could stop them. I'm reminded of the joke about the man who is in a near fatal car accident and is on his way to the hospital with sirens screaming. With his wife holding his hand, he opens one eye and asks, "Is there time for a quickie?" Although we joke about constant erections, the truth is erections are complex and easily can become disrupted, particularly as men age.

Is Osteoporosis a Problem for Men Going through Male Menopause?

According to most information available on osteoporosis, it is a bone disease that affects women. Dr. Robert Lindsay, M.D., Ph.D., and president of the National Osteoporosis Foundation, says that a majority of the one thousand men recently questioned by a Gallup survey believed they could not have osteoporosis. However, Dr. Eric Orwoll, a leading medical researcher in the field of osteoporosis in men says that 1.5 million men have osteoporosis and another 3.5 million are at high risk. American men over fifty years of age have a higher risk of suffering an osteo-related fracture than developing clinical prostate cancer. One-third of the men who suffer hip fracture will die within a year.

Men of all ethnic groups are affected, however, white men appear to be at the greatest risk for osteoporosis.

What Can a Man Do to Prevent Osteoporosis?

Educate yourself and as soon as possible begin preventative actions to "head off" this disease. Know whether or not you are at risk and take action. Visit with your private physician about whether or not he feels you are at risk and need to be tested. The sooner an individual begins preventative measures, the better.

If you smoke, stop.

Get regular exercise.

Get proper amounts of calcium—recommended to be 1000 mg/day for adults—the best sources are skim milk and nonfat yogurt. Adequate Vitamin D, B6, B12, and K are also important. Some recommendations are for 1500 mg/day of calcium for sixty-five-year-old males. Get as much of the above recommended vitamins through diet and then supplement. The National Osteoporosis Foundation recommends TUMS as an excellent calcium source.

Limit alcohol intake.

Chapter 3

———

Manhood—
The Big Impossible?

How to Survive
Adolescence and Middlescence

Though I hadn't seen my father since he had his midlife breakdown and left when I was five, we reconnected in the last ten years of his life. He lived to be ninety. He loved baseball and used it as a metaphor for life. He said, you have to keep coming up to the plate no matter how many times you strike out and you only win by getting around all three bases and touching home plate.

I often thought about his baseball analogy when I contemplated my life and the life of many men I know and work with. If second base is midlife, I believe men are dropping out at three places. Too many young men never make it to first. Their philosophy seems to be "live fast, die young." They end up in prison, on drugs, or dead on the streets.

Other men are afraid of getting old. They become obsessed with youth and beauty. These are the guys who leave their partners for someone younger and prettier. They are afraid to make the turn toward home, run on past second, and end up alone in left field.

A third group makes the turn at second, but sees the second half of life as a time of increasing loss. I call them the downhill cynics. They expect to deteriorate, to get old and sick. I see them going past third and ending up dead in the dugout.

The key to success, as my father said, was to make it around all three bases and get home safely, perhaps then to become a "coach" and help others make the journey successfully.

In order to understand the male menopause journey and what lies ahead in the second half of life, we need to take a tour through the male life cycle to help us understand what it means to be a man.

Seasons of a Man's Life

Erik H. Erikson was a Pulitzer prize–winning author and one of the leading figures in the field of psychology and human development. One of his finest achievements was to develop a model called the Eight Stages of Man that looked at human developments through the life cycle. The model suggests that at each stage there are two crucial dimensions, one that signals a successful completion and one that suggests an unsuccessful one.

Infancy I: Basic Trust vs. Basic Mistrust

The first demonstration of social trust in the baby is the ease of his feeding, the depth of his sleep, and the relaxation of his bowels. A great deal of success at this stage depends on a loving and consistent relationship with the mother.

Infancy II: Autonomy vs. Shame and Doubt

This is a period when the infant/child deals with two skills, holding on and letting go. At this stage, the infant reaches out more to the world and begins to get a sense of rightness about his actions or comes to doubt and feel ashamed of himself.

Shame is expressed early in an impulse to bury one's face, or to sink into the ground and disappear forever.

Many adults, trying to control a child's behavior, end up making the child feel ashamed. Shaming, rather than helping a child learn socially acceptable behavior, leads to a secret determination to try and get away with things, to be defiant, and to do anything he can to rebel.

At midlife, men often have to deal with the shame that they still carry from their early life experiences.

Childhood I: Initiative vs. Guilt

At this stage, the child is walking and is becoming more his own person. He possesses a surplus of energy which enables him to go after things he wants even if there is danger involved. He may become aggressive with siblings or others. He needs boundaries from parents without being made to feel guilty for his aggressive feelings or his childhood sexuality, which begins to emerge at this stage.

If the child is made to feel guilty about his desires, the feelings go underground and a tremendous amount of rage may develop as some of the child's fondest hopes and wildest fantasies are inhibited.

Again, as in the previous stages, these repressed desires often surface again in menopausal men, which, if not understood, can cause tremendous harm to the man and his family.

Childhood II: Industry vs. Inferiority

The child now enters the life of the schoolroom. He must forget past hopes and wishes, while his exuberant imagination is tamed and harnessed to the unnatural rhythms of school. This seems particularly difficult for more physical and active boys who must sit still rather than move about. If they continue their activity, many are mistakenly labeled as troublemakers or having attention deficit disorder and treated rather than understood.

Many boys often come to feel inferior which can lead to school dropout, a lowering of self-esteem, or a make-believe personality that appears to get along, but harbors great resentment and anger.

Adolescence and Puberty: Identity vs. Role Confusion

With the advent of puberty, childhood comes to an end and youth begins. At this stage of life, all the integration that has taken place in childhood is shaken up as hormones begin to assert themselves and physical, psychological, interpersonal, sexual, social, and spiritual changes begin to occur.

Up until this point in the life cycle, boys and girls have been quite similar in the way they move through each stage. With the advent of puberty and the surge of testosterone, things change dramatically. As Michael Gurian, author of *The Wonder of Boys*, says, "When a boy hits puberty, the influence of testosterone on the brain increases manifold. His testosterone level itself will increase in quantities ten to twenty times more than girls. His genitals will increase to eight times their previous size. His body will process anywhere between five to seven surges of testosterone per day. You can expect him to masturbate continually, bump into things a lot, be moody and aggressive, require a great deal of sleep, lose his temper, want sex as soon as he gets up the emotional guts to propose to a partner, and have a massive sexual fantasy life."

As we will see, there are major similarities between what goes on in puberty and what goes on in male menopause. In both cases, males are searching for an identity amid the changes that can bring out so much role confusion.

Adulthood I: Intimacy vs. Isolation

The strength acquired at each stage is tested in the next. When a man feels his identity is strong, he wants to test it out by reaching out for the intimacy he gets when connecting to another person. The counterpart to intimacy is isolation, which men who have not adequately completed other stages often experience.

Sigmund Freud, the father of psychoanalysis, was once asked what a normal person should be able to do. His answer was short and sweet. "Lieben und arbeiten" (To love and to work), he said. It's a simple formula and Freud offers us five guidelines for health at this stage of life:

1. Mutual sexual satisfaction
2. With a loved partner
3. With whom one is able and willing to share a mutual trust.
4. And with whom one is able and willing to regulate the cycles of
   a. work
   b. procreation
   c. recreation
5. So as to secure to any children the couple brings into the world, all the stages of a satisfactory development that will allow the children to grow up healthy and joyful.

It would be wonderful if life worked this simply, but it's nice to know how things could work if we were successful at each stage of the life cycle.

Adulthood II: Generativity vs. Stagnation

This is the stage that male menopause prepares a man to engage. If the previous stage focuses on love and work and can help the individual, couple, and their family to grow and prosper, this stage speaks more to the bigger picture. The previous stage recognizes that it takes a healthy mother and father to raise a child. This stage recognizes that it takes a "village" to insure that the mothers and fathers of the world have the support they need to raise the children of the world.

Whether a man has children of his own or not, he often feels a need to feel productive and creative in helping all children, in making the world a safer place for children. This is the stage I call "Super-Adulthood" and it requires a man to step up to the plate and become a super man, a hero to the young fathers who need his support in order to raise the young children well. If he doesn't engage this stage in a positive way, he begins to stagnate and go downhill, physically, emotionally, and spiritually.

This is why we see so many men in these middle years, between forty and fifty-five, acting like aging children. They either become sick and need to be taken care of like a child or they are out buying themselves the latest gadgets and toys.

What they need is to be able to find a way to give to others in a meaningful way. They need to feel that they are needed and they have something significant to offer their families, their communities, and the world.

Independence Day: If I'd Only Known about Male Menopause Sooner

Last July 4th, Independence Day, my husband of thirty-three years left me for another woman. He was fifty-five and I was fifty-one. He told me he had found someone else who was more fun and wanted to do all the things he wanted to do. He was very cruel and spared no one, not even our three grown children or three grandchildren.

He said everything was our fault, and still is, that we drove him to it and he tried to warn us all. The repercussions of what occurred after that event were devastating to the entire family, emotionally, financially, physically, and spiritually.

Our family fell apart. He walked away from a business he had started several years ago with our sons and totally cut off all communications with anyone in the family except for an occasional call to our daughter who is torn and constantly in tears because of what her father has done.

I only wish I could have learned about male menopause sooner. You see, for the past two years he has had all the symptoms mentioned in your book. I had no idea what was going on. He kept complaining about being so lonely, even though I was always there for him. I knew how he felt about his looks and his idea of staying "forever young." He bought a new Harley, but it was never fast enough, and he went to Sturgis for the bike rallies, but it didn't seem to satisfy him as it once had.

This is where he met his new love. I truly thought we had a good marriage and loved each other. We had been through so much together over the years. I was hoping the future would be easier and more comfortable for us. The kids were gone and we were finally free. But he said he didn't want to spend his time baby-sitting the grandchildren, that he had his life to live.

In his eyes, I became boring, fat, slept too much, and certainly not the image with which he wanted to fulfill his new dream. It was over that fast. We are now divorced.

I've been through so much heartbreak and pain, at times I never thought I'd live through it. Who is this man that I married and loved for so many years? No one knows him anymore, not even his own children.

Unfortunately, we have two sons that are described perfectly in your book. One who was shamed and turned to drugs and the other who doesn't think he's worth anything because he spent his whole life trying to make his dad happy, and now feels he's somehow failed because his dad left.

We will pick up the pieces and be a family again, but I cannot express to you, after reading your first book, "If I had only known." I still love him very much. I don't even know what happened to him and to us, it all took place so fast. He severed the ties the only way he knew how, brutally.

As the Christmas holidays approach, we are all fumbling with emotions. No one said life is fair, but to be this cruel is almost unforgivable and I'm not sure the children will ever forgive their father. What makes a man throw away his whole life—all he's worked for and nurtured—for a chance at being an adolescent again? I finally have come to know the answer—male menopause.

As I read your book, over and over I would say to myself, yes, this is him, this is him, this is him. I wanted to scream it to the world. I wanted to scream it at him. I look at men in a different way now and almost feel sad for them. I still love him and wish he would still hear my plea. "Don't give up on us, don't give up on yourself, don't give up on our family."

June

Points of understanding:

• One of the keys to understanding male menopause is that it relates to a desire for men to find their freedom, to break away from the life of first adulthood and capture a new life. It is similar to adolescence when boys rebel and turn away from family members and those they love.

• If early symptoms are not recognized, the pressure builds up. Often, the younger woman is seen as the symbol of the new life and their "old lady" symbolizes the past life they are growing away from. Dramatic, often destructive action results when we don't understand what is going on.

• Not only does the action affect the man and the woman, but grown children also are impacted. They blame themselves or their fathers for changes they don't understand.

• The answer to the pain of so many is to understand male menopause and to prevent major problems before they occur. Holding this book, I know you are on this path. It is a path that will require the very best of you. Stick with it. Those who have gone before will light the way.

I Convinced Him He Is Going through Male Menopause

After twenty-eight years of marriage, my husband said, "I don't love you anymore." He said that life is passing him by; the children don't need him now that they're grown, and he feels he needs something new. Sound familiar? He behaved exactly like the men you describe. Fortunately for me, he agreed to read your book. I was able to convince him that he is going through male menopause. He truly related to what you said.

We spent hours going through the book together. I didn't talk much, just listened to him as he told me the hopes, fears, and worries he was experiencing. After weeks of talking, he finally broke down and cried. It was the first time he had cried since his mother died.

I told him that I wanted to support his need for freedom and his desire to make changes in his life, but I also loved and needed him. Even though the children are grown, I know they need him, too.

He had been traveling a lot for the past three years. He liked to be on his own, but had become isolated from us. He felt that the job really needed him, but we didn't.

With a better understanding of what he is going through, he apologized to the children and to me. He said that he had "lost it" and he was really sorry. We're now working to restore our relationship on a new, and hopefully stronger, footing.

Marla

Points of understanding:

• Every man goes through male menopause differently, just like every boy goes through adolescence differently. Both have great difficulty talking about what is really going on inside.

• Many men feel that they are no longer needed. As the roles they had as younger men change, they have not learned new roles and often feel lost.

• Women often want to reassure their partners that they are loved and appreciated. What men need more than anything is just to be listened to, not to be "helped."

• As their families become more independent, men wonder what they really have to offer. The things that they had given in the past are no longer necessary, but they haven't developed their new talents and gifts yet. Both the man and the woman need to search together for what they each have to offer themselves and their families in the second half of life.

Mature Adulthood: Ego Integrity vs. Despair

This is the stage of life where we can pull things together and feel that our lives have made sense, that we have given to ourselves and others and have made the world a little better place.

It is a stage of personal acceptance where a man can look back at his triumphs and failures and recognize that all parts were important, that he needed to experience it all.

The lack or loss of this sense of integrity is signified by fear of death. Despair expresses the feeling that a man has failed to live up to the best of what he could be, to become his own man. He feels that time is running out and it's too late to start another life and try out alternate roads to personal integrity.

There is an old story about a Jewish rabbi that illustrates the importance of finding and keeping our sense of self. "When I get to heaven," said the Hasidic rabbi Susya shortly before his death, "they will not ask me, 'Why were you not Moses?' but, 'Why were you not Susya? Why did you not become what only you could become?'"

Although it is the most difficult task of all, it is really quite simple. All we are asked to do is become ourselves, to live our own lives with integrity.

This brings our life cycle full circle. We see there is a relationship between the first value, trust, with the last value, integrity. "Healthy children will not fear life," says Erikson, "if their elders have integrity enough not to fear death."

Although these stages fit both males and females, we will see in future chapters that there are differences in the ways that males and females experience them. The most significant changes occur during adolescence and middlescence.

Adolescence and Middlescence

Author Gail Sheehy says, "Middlescence is adolescence the second time around. Turning backward, going around in circles, feeling lost in a buzz of confusion and unable to make decisions."

Does this sound familiar? What are we seeing?

• Mood swings

• Hormonal shifts

• Confusion about sexuality

• Desire to break away from family and at the same time clinging tightly to family for support

• Obsession with the latest toys and gadgets

• Need for intimacy and fears of getting close

• Physical changes in the body

• Questions about identity and direction in life

I think we all recognize these signs. But are we looking at a fifteen-year-old or a fifty-year-old? The truth is we are looking at both. Adolescence and middlescence are very similar stages in life. It's one of the reasons that midlife parents have such a difficult time dealing with their teenage kids—they are both dealing with the same issues. When Dad freaks out thinking about his daughter's emerging sexuality, it is often because he is also dealing with changes in his own sexuality. When father has difficulty setting reasonable limits on his son's behavior, it is often because he is having trouble setting limits for himself.

I Feel Like I'm a Teenager Again

I am forty-four and have experienced a lot of the changes already. Your book helped me understand them even more. I also realize I'm not alone.

Last winter, I went through a huge change. I think it was triggered by fights I was having with my teenage son. His behavior was becoming more and more intolerable. He wasn't coming home at night, refusing to listen to me or his mother, and fighting whenever

I tried to discipline him. He seemed totally out of control. I felt like hitting him. We finally decided to try family counseling which led to individual counseling for me. It has made all the difference in the world.

I realize now I was feeling the same fearful, angry, and depressive emotions I felt at a very young age in the military. At first I thought it might be post-traumatic stress disorder or something like that. I finally let it all out with the counselor. It felt great to let out long-buried emotions and experiences I hadn't told anyone. The counselor helped me work through a lot of it.

I've been working with amateur boxers since I got out of the military and it helps me to pass on my knowledge to younger men. I saw that a lot of their young male energy was triggering my own feelings. It was like reliving my own adolescence, but not being aware of it. I thought I'd grown out of that when I went into the service when I was eighteen.

Recently I've seen the movie *Saving Private Ryan*. I am hearing from other veterans that it triggered a lot of feelings that they had never let out before. I'm seeing how many, like me, didn't seek professional counseling and are going through emotional stress many years later. As you said, if you don't deal with life changes when they come along, they are much worse later.

I didn't have trouble dealing with the movie, thanks to the counseling help I've received and from the support I got reading your book. Hopefully, we will deal more directly with male menopause in the future. We badly need to understand that women are not the only ones who have emotional and physical changes at midlife.

The winters here are a true test of tolerance for depression. Last year I finally came to grips with a lot of that.

I've begun doing many of the things you mentioned in your book including joining a men's group, changing my diet, exercising, as well as cutting down on my alcohol consumption.

When I was younger, I made the mistake of dealing with anger and fear by drinking my way through life. There wasn't professional help available for me back then, like there is now, so I played hell with myself for many years. There were a lot of very bad and unlucky years in my life and I had a really rough time dealing with it.

My life has improved significantly in the last few years, more like coming to grips with solving problems the right way.

Anyway, as I talk to more and more guys my age going through the same things, they really don't want to come to grips with it or don't know how. There is a lot of fear. I advise them to read your book and seek some good counseling.

For some reason, men suffer with the "real man syndrome" where they feel they don't need anyone's help, which is not good at all.

Hopefully as more of us deal with male menopause we can look forward to a better second half of life.

Alex

Points of understanding:

• Quite often, the issues of middlescence are triggered by those of adolescence. A son or a daughter begins to act out and it becomes clear that there are significant family problems.

• It is quite rare for a man to recognize that the problem is not the fault of the adolescent but involves the whole family. And it is even rarer to recognize that he might need some counseling for himself.

• As a man looks within, particularly with the help of a real confidant or counselor, he begins to let out long-buried pain and shame that had been covered over for a long time.

• Movies, old songs, pictures, etc., often trigger old memories that must now be dealt with more directly.

• There is a lot of misunderstanding and fear about this time of life and most men want to avoid it if possible. It is often helpful to get support from other men who are going through the same things.

• Dealing directly with depression and cutting back or stopping alcohol consumption are often very helpful decisions for men to make as they deal with their physical and emotional health.

• Many men suffer from the belief that asking for help or admitting weakness is a sign that they are not "real" men. In fact, the opposite is true. It takes a real man, a brave man, a man of integrity, to ask for help. Any man can suffer in silence. We've been trained to do that since we were boys. Reaching out to others takes real courage.

• Just as young males need the support of older males when going through adolescence, midlife men also need the support of older men in order to successfully complete middlescence and move into the next stage of manhood.

Manhood: The Big Impossible

In the first cross-cultural study of manhood, anthropologist David Gilmore found that becoming a man is a process that must be achieved through a series of tests that a boy must complete successfully in order to be perceived by himself and his community as a man.

Among the Fox tribe of Iowa, for example, being a man does not come easily. Based on stringent standards of accomplishment in tribal affairs and economic pursuits, real manhood is said to be the "Big Impossible," an exclusive status that only a nimble few can achieve.

Gilmore found that in cultures as diverse as those of Japan, India, China, the Mediterranean, aboriginal South America, Oceania, East Africa, ancient Greece, and modern North America, the pattern was similar.

Boys cannot become men except through a rite of passage. "Masculinity is not something given to you, something you're born with," says author Norman Mailer, "but something you gain.…And you gain it by winning small battles of honor."

Although there are rites for initiating girls into womanhood, there is no parallel cross-cultural belief that girls have to be *made* into women. In all cultures Gilmore studied, womanhood is seen as developing naturally, needing no cultural intervention, its predestined arrival at menarche commemorated, rather than forced by ritual.

There is a primal insecurity that males experience about being men that I have not found with females. A woman may ask herself if she is being a good enough mother, wife, or friend. But rarely does she question her identity as a woman. For males this is not the case. There is continuous questioning.

The insecurity stems from four sources:

1. As a child, he comes to realize that his primary love object, his mother, is different from him. He will never grow up to be like her. I saw a young toddler proclaim with pride, "When I grow up I'm going to have a baby." When told by his mother, "No, only girls can have babies," he burst into tears.

2. The love object that he is supposed to identify with is often absent physically or emotionally. As boys, we hunger for our fathers and for the parts of ourselves that only our father's presence can bring out in us.

Poet Robert Bly says, "When a father and son spend long hours together, we could say that a substance almost like food passes from the older body to the younger body." Without that nourishment we starve.

I hear so many men at midlife begin to feel the grief when they come to grips with the fact that they never really knew their fathers. "The son does not receive a hands-on healing, but a body-on healing," says Bly. "His cells receive some knowledge of what an adult masculine body is. The young man comes to learn the sound that male cells sing."

What would we give to know our fathers so well that our cells vibrated in unison? How sweet would it be to know the sound that male cells sing? How many lifetimes have we been searching for the nutrients that would nourish us and validate our manhood as sons of our fathers? I shiver with sadness when I say these words out loud. It's no wonder that so many men feel a grief beyond imagining and a rage that knows no bounds.

Single Mothers with Sons Truly Need This Information

I can't begin to tell you the impact your book has had on me. Initially, I thought I'd read it to better understand what men experience. I grew up without a father, as my parents divorced when I was quite young, and I realized my information is limited.

However, I did not realize that you would address an issue crucial to me at this point in my life—my son. I feel quite emotional about just writing this. I raised my son, now eighteen, since he was three years old. His father chose to spend little or no time at all with him.

About two years ago, Jordan began to have noticeable difficulty with anger. His anger escalated into rage on many occasions, culminating last November with violence.

I knew Jordan needed a male role model, but I didn't know what to do. I just didn't realized how absolutely crucial it was for him. Now I understand. I can see, as never before, the effect that his father's leaving has had on his life.

There were parts of your book that affected me so deeply, I cried. This was really healthy. I now have information I was never before provided. When you wrote about your experience at the men's retreat when you finally confronted your feelings about your mother and the relationship you had with her, I was truly shaken.

Single mothers with boys truly need your information.

Casandra

Points of understanding:

• Most men and women don't truly comprehend how important fathers are in the lives of their children. When a father leaves, the wound seems to heal and life goes on. It's often in adolescence that the depth of the pain becomes obvious. Women often take the brunt of the boy's anger at having been abandoned.

• Every effort should be made to work through differences and keep families intact. Failing that, every effort should be made to keep fathers involved in the raising of their children.

3. No matter how much we would like to feel we are part of the mystery of new life, there is always some insecurity. Whether a woman actually has children or not, she knows that her body is made to carry a baby inside. A male's contribution of sperm, though essential, does not give the same feeling of pride that the knowledge you can carry a baby, birth it, and nourish it, offers.

Men may seek to compensate in many ways. We can make lots of money, build skyscrapers, go to the moon. But it doesn't look like anytime soon we will have the same intimate relationship to new life that a woman has.

And even if we manage to find a woman who wants to mate with us and she gets pregnant, we are never 100 percent sure that the child is ours. From a biological point of view, success is defined by the degree to which your genes make it into future generations. Every woman who gets pregnant knows that the child carries her genes. Every man, no matter how sure he is of his fatherhood, must always harbor some degree of doubt. He can never be totally sure if some other man's sperm may have gotten there first. "Simply put, children are inescapably 'Mommy's babies, Daddy's maybes,'" say David P. Barash, Ph.D., and Judith Eve Lipton, M.D., authors of *Making Sense of Sex.* "Whereas every mother naturally bears an ironclad relationship to her child, no father can be entirely confident—short of keeping his wife in solitary confinement, shackling her with a chastity belt, or demanding DNA testing—that he is the real (that is, the genetic) father."

4. Boys need a rite of passage led by the elder males in the community that allows the young men to test themselves and, if

successful, to be accepted by the larger community. Without this direction, young men try, unsuccessfully, to initiate themselves. This accounts, I believe, for a lot of the gang membership and violence we see in the society. Males also need an initiation into second adulthood. Without this initiation, older men cannot become the elders that the society needs.

These factors help account for the reason men are generally insecure. They help us understand the higher level of sexual insecurity and jealousy men experience, as well as their willingness to become violent more easily or put themselves in dangerous situations.

When you don't feel like a man inside, you are always trying to show the world that you really *are* the man you are pretending to be. Probably the truest statement of how cut off men really are from their true natures was given by Eugene O'Neil in the play *Long Day's Journey into Night*:

> It was a great mistake, my being born a man. I would have been much more successful as a sea gull or a fish. As it is, I will always be a stranger who never feels at home, who does not really want and is not really wanted, who can never belong, who must always be a little in love with death!

Rites of Passage and Validation of a Male Ally

There are two things a man needs to overcome his insecurity and fear and to take his place as a man among men. The first is a rite of passage from adolescence to adulthood and from middlescence to what I call super-adulthood. The second is the involvement, at key times of his life, of a male ally.

What is a rite of passage? Anthropologist Mircea Eliade defines it this way: "Rites of passage are a category of rituals that mark the passage of a person through the life cycle, from one stage to another over time, from one role or social position to another."

We can think of a rite of passage as a forced journey through a rocky canyon so hard and narrow that you can't take your baggage with you. Within the ritual of the rite we are given the opportunity to face our emotional and experiential limitations and to move beyond them.

The initiate often experiences a "second birth." They "die" in one phase of their lives and the roles associated with that period, leaving it behind, and enter a new stage with new identity.

Ours is one of the few cultures in human history that does not incorporate rites of passage into the lives of its members. It is a failing that is costly to the young men as well as the society at large. This is now beginning to change. "Over the last decade, models of initiation have been created by people all over North America," says Michael Gurian, author of *The Wonder of Boys.*

It is the community of elders in a society that provides the structure and direction for the rites of passage which are particularly necessary for young boys. Malidoma Some, himself an initiated elder, says, "Elders and mentors have an irreplaceable function in the life of any community. Without them, the young are lost—their overflowing energies wasted in useless pursuits. The old must live in the young like a grounding force that tames the tendency towards bold but senseless actions and shows them the path of wisdom. In the absence of elders, the impetuosity of youth becomes the slow death of the community."

I was fortunate that as a young man I stumbled into a community that took rites of passage seriously. On the surface, it was an unlikely place for a young man to get support and nurturing. The place was called Synanon, a treatment program that used direct confrontation to help addicts recover and live healthy lives again. It was the place where I received my initiation from adolescence into manhood. It took place over a period of five years from the time I was nineteen until I was twenty-four.

Like all true initiations, this one can't be put into words. I can give you some feeling for the process and the elder who lead the initiation.

When I first got involved with Synanon, I was terrified and confused, but I kept up the appearance of a self-assured young graduate student who knew exactly what he wanted and where he was going.

Though I wasn't aware of it at the time, I think I joined Synanon because I hoped they might look below the surface and see the lost child I was hiding. Maybe they would force me to do what I didn't feel I could do myself—help me drop my mask and help me develop the courage to let others know me—to finally become a man. As I signed up for my first Synanon "game," I thought of the words my mother had written in my fourth grade autograph book. Quoting Shakespeare's Hamlet she told me: "This above all: To thine own self be true, And it must follow, as the night the day, Thou canst not then be false to any man."

I always felt those words held the key to my life, but I had no idea how to put them into practice. How did I go about finding my true self? If I did find it would people really want to know it? The few times I had let the real me out to my mother, it was clear that there were only certain parts of the real me that she was comfortable with: anger, sexual desire, and a fierce need for independence clearly weren't acceptable.

It was in the small group sessions, the Synanon games, that I began to learn the tools of self-knowledge and self-care. Before each session of the Synanon game, someone would read the Synanon Philosophy. Based on the writings of Ralph Waldo Emerson, it gave me a structure to guide my search for self. Thirty-five years later, I still remember the first lines:

> The Synanon Philosophy is based on the belief that there comes a time in everyone's life when he arrives at the conviction that envy is ignorance; that imitation is suicide; that he must accept himself for better or for worse as is his portion; that though the wide universe is full of good, no kernel of nourishing corn can come to him but through his toil bestowed on that plot of ground which is given to him to till.

Each time I heard the philosophy I thought of the evening I had first met Chuck Dederich. Dederich started Synanon in 1958 in Ocean Park, California, with a $33 unemployment check. By the time I got involved in 1965, Synanon had grown to become a multimillion-dollar corporation helping thousands of addicts.

Dederich was a controversial figure, a man who had dreams of saving the world by creating a community of men and women who could heal from drug addiction, a disease that was thought at the time to be incurable. He was called by various people a madman, a saint, an opportunist, a brilliant executive, a latter-day Socrates, an earthquake, a herd of one elephant. Chuck was my first ally.

For me, the word "ally" suggests someone who is compassionate, friendly, and helpful. There is a gentleness and kindness implied. But ally also brings to mind the warrior energy of men who support each other under fire, who can be passionate, flinty, and courageous.

I remember Chuck talking about the Synanon game, the core group experience of the community that helped addicts find their way back to themselves. I was mesmerized. It felt like he was talking just to me: "Some young guy will come to me and say, 'Chuck, what'll I do? I'm frantic, I'm desperate!' And I'll say, 'Lad, go find yourself!' And he'll say, 'Oh, gee, thanks. That's great…' And he walks out of the office door and…what in the hell's he do? Does he start looking around the stairway or over his shoulder or what? What in the name of God does it mean: 'George, go find yourself'?"

As I listened, I felt I was going to get some practical knowledge that Shakespeare couldn't give, but that this ex-drunk from Toledo, Ohio, could offer me.

"In Synanon," Dederich went on, "there is provided an opportunity to open the door. It's a key to the room where you are; the room that life has locked you in to where you can't find yourself. You stand outside the door, or outside the room—sometimes you don't even know where the door is—and there you are…in there. You can't find yourself."

As I listened to Dederich's words, I felt he understood my confusion and fear. He seemed to know what it was like to go through life, trying to be someone else, because I didn't have a clue about how to find my true self.

"In Synanon we have found the key. We know that if you take this key in your hot little hand and insert it into the lock and twist hard enough, that door will open. The door will open a little at a time and you'll begin to find yourself. You'll get a glimpse, at first. Then more will be revealed as time goes on."

I was ready to take the key and open the door. I was anxious to know how playing the Synanon game would help me open the door to my true self. Dederich had an answer that was so simple and direct I couldn't believe it would work until I tried it.

"Here's the key: If you're a tantrum-thrower, a guy who loves being the center of attention, then by all means make every effort you can to do it well...for awhile. But then, for heaven's sake, start doing yourself a favor. Sit back and listen to others. Just sit there. Keep your mouth shut. I'll tell you something...you're not going to believe it because you won't believe it until you've had the experience. You won't die. You really won't, you know. And you might just begin to find out about who you are under all of that bluster.

"And you people on the other end of the stick. You know who you are." When Dederich's gaze fell on me, I swallowed hard. "You people who tend to be somewhat passive and seek the dark corners of the room, you know who I'm talking to. You'll do anything to melt into the background and keep from calling attention to yourselves. Well, by all means be a good wallflower, for awhile. But then learn to get into the fray, roll up your sleeves and learn to spit out some real good invective at a tyrant. What the hell's the difference who. We're all tyrants sometimes and we all need to stand up against the bullies of the world."

I realized I was beginning to understand how to use the key. I had to practice doing something which at first seemed like a violation of my very being. To be the center of attention, to raise my voice, to stand up and fight for what I believed in, was terrifying. In my family you just didn't do that. But I found out that I needed to allow the hidden to emerge if I was going to learn who I was and what it meant to find myself.

The Synanon game was the place where I began to learn how to tell the truth and speak from my heart. I remember the first time I felt comfortable raising my voice and screaming at a woman who was trying to make me feel guilty for not being a good enough son to my parents.

I remember the first time I could say "fuck you" out loud and not feel ashamed.

I remember refusing to go along with Synanon and sell fight tickets because I didn't believe in violence. For months I was "attacked" in the games and learned how to stand up for my convictions.

It didn't occur to me at the time, but the "attacks" were actually offered with love. They weren't meant to beat me into submission, but rather to force me to own my own strength. Once I defended my position long enough that I was convinced I was right, the attacks stopped.

My initiation came to an end when I decided to start a treatment program for addicts at a local hospital. This time I was mercilessly attacked for trying to do a job that was way over my head. "Who the hell do you think you are," someone would scream at me in the game. "Haven't you learned anything here? Don't you know Synanon is the only program that can help an addict. You're killing people!"

I defended myself as best I could. I thought I could do something good at the hospital, but I also wondered if they were right. Who the hell was I really to think I could take on a man's job?

For months, I was forced to face the onslaught at every game I was in. I wasn't sure how long I could last. One day, Dederich came into my group, and I felt my blood turn to ice. I was terrified of what he would say to me and how I would stand up to his questioning of my abilities.

When it was my turn to come under his scrutiny, he fixed me with a stare that pinned me to the wall. "I heard of you," he roared. I imagined I could feel the walls shake. "You're the youngster who thinks he's going to save addicts. Is that right?" My knees really did feel like rubber and my throat would barely open. I wanted to run, but I looked him in the eye and answered. "Yeah, Chuck, I think I'm doing the right thing."

Dederich's gaze was intense and I shivered. Then he cracked a smile, shaking his head. "I do believe you just might be. Keep up the good work, son. Someday you're going to be running that hospital." I never ran the hospital, but I always felt that Chuck believed I could.

"Younger men need the blessing of older men if they are to feel empowered in the world," says psychologist Robert Moore. The blessing I received from Chuck in those few moments will last my whole life.

Those lucky enough to have had an adolescent initiation will find it easier to recognize the need at midlife. For those who did not have one, the midlife initiation is even more crucial.

Male Menopause and the Midlife Initiation

Since we live in a culture where formal initiations are rare, most initiations happen by accident. Many are triggered by a major life event, seemingly out of our control. It could be a divorce, loss of a job, death of a parent, mental illness in a family member, or a personal brush with mortality.

At midlife, there is often an event that begins male menopause. Like the adolescent rite of passage, it is meant to force us to let go of our past and move ahead to the future. The harder we hang on to the past, the more difficult this passage becomes. What follows is a description of my own initiation.

The beginning of my own rite of passage was both subtle and dramatic. The drama began when I got the call from my doctor. "Jed, we've got the results of your tests and I'd like to see you in my office as soon as possible." Dr. Volen's voice was calm. My heart seemed to stop, then tried to escape through my throat.

Just moments before the attack that had sent me to the doctor for tests, I was on top of the world. I was forty-seven years old, had just signed a major book contract, was traveling all over the country giving workshops and lectures, and was happily married and looking forward to more time with my wife now that our last two children had left home.

Feeling more physically fit than I ever had, I was doing my daily three-mile run. The sky was sparkling blue and the summer heat caused a satisfying sweat to cover my body. Suddenly, my heart began pounding wildly and my head felt like it was about to explode. The pain brought me to my knees and I sat on the ground stunned and shaken.

Within hours, however, the pain had disappeared and I felt like my old self. I decided to ignore whatever it was, figured I was fine, and kept the experience to myself. I didn't want to worry my wife.

From the time I was a little boy, I learned to ignore pain, that boys don't cry or complain, and you don't ask for help unless you're bleeding to death. The next day, however, I had another attack. Something was happening that I couldn't ignore.

Even seated in the doctor's office, I was sure the concern was unwarranted until he gave me the news. "The tests indicate that you've got an adrenal tumor," the doctor said looking me straight in the eye. "It will need to come out as soon as possible." I couldn't believe what I was hearing. I couldn't have a tumor. I was too young. I was too healthy. I was doing all the right things. There must be some mistake. But there wasn't, and the surgery proceeded. I survived and life went on, though it was never the same. Having been close to death, I appreciated life in a new way.

The other changes were less dramatic. They nibbled at the edges of my consciousness, easier to push away, but like mosquitoes at nightfall, they were more pesky and persistent. My mother had died when I was forty-three and since then thoughts about death found their way into my awareness at the most unexpected times.

Even though our three oldest children were grown, I now found myself worrying about whether they would make it. The world seemed so much more chaotic and dangerous than when I left for college at age seventeen.

I felt finished with the day-to-day responsibilities of raising children, but was concerned about the increasing levels of violence, particularly among young males, in our society. Young men seemed to need the guidance of older males. Was I ready to be one of those "older males?" Having grown up without the presence of a father, I was afraid that there was some critical male wisdom I had never gotten myself and so would not be able to pass on to my sons.

My work was OK but I wondered whether there was more I should be doing. Is this the way I wanted to spend the rest of my life? I didn't feel passionate about my work as I once had, but I had no idea what else I might do.

I felt restless and irritable. I wanted to do something new, but I had no idea what it might be. My friends suddenly seemed less interesting. It didn't seem like we had much in common and they often appeared immature and foolish. They were never available when I needed them and were always in my face when I wanted to be alone.

I was a city boy, born in New York, raised in Los Angeles, and living near San Francisco. I loved the urban diversity and excitement, but had fantasies of living in the country where things were slower and quieter.

Things with my wife were good, yet I felt uneasy and confused. I had expected that when the kids were gone we would be closer, more intimate, and would finally have more time for each other, more time for sex. But just when I seemed to want to move in, her energy was moving outward. She wanted to start a school, teach classes, travel. I wanted to stay at home more and "cocoon." It wasn't the easy time I had expected.

I often blamed her for not being there when I needed her, not wanting me, not making our relationship a priority in our lives. She complained that I was irritated and angry most of the time. She closed down when I'd strike out in anger. We were caught in a horrible downward spiral. I'd tell her the reason I was so angry was that she was withdrawing from me. She'd respond by telling me she withdrew to protect herself from my anger.

I knew I was stuck and needed a new rite of passage to help me through male menopause. I contacted a friend who was the head of New Warriors (now called the ManKind Project).

The twin goals of the organization offered me a new focus and seemed to be the kind of midlife initiation I was looking to experience. The first goal is to initiate men into a mature masculinity, to lead lives of integrity, to connect with feelings, and to renew responsibility for their personal mission in the world. The second goal is to be of service to the community, both as individual men with a reinvigorated sense of compassion and personal responsibility, and as communities of men who share a close-knit bond.

Once again, I prepared myself. The initiation culminated with a weekend experience that fulfilled its promise as a true rite of passage. It was transformative, a celebration of manhood, and an opportunity to fully develop our life purpose.

The day after I returned from the New Warriors weekend, I got a call from my nineteen-year-old stepson, Aaron. As we talked about what was going on in our lives, he seemed down and I was overflowing with my experience. "I've never heard you so enthusiastic about anything before," he told me over the phone.

"You've done a lot of men's events. If your experience was that good, I want to go." As luck, or the workings of the gods, would have it, there was a new center opening up in Portland, Oregon, where

Aaron lived. Aaron was accepted to be part of the next weekend initiation and I was allowed to participate on staff.

Watching my son be mentored by older men and participating with him in his own rite of passage was one of the most moving and valuable experiences of my life. If my own weekend helped me feel the power of initiation, to feel deeply accepted as a man, the weekend with Aaron helped me recognize how important older men are in the lives of younger men.

Aaron and I had inherited each other when Carlin and I got together. He already had a father and I already had children and the nature of this "step" relationship wasn't clear. In my tentative way, I tried to be a supportive presence in Aaron's life without going over the line and being intrusive. I didn't want to replace his father or get in the way of his relationship with his mother.

During the weekend, more happened than I could begin to share, but in a very emotional encounter, Aaron told me honestly that he felt I had failed him as a father. "I wanted more of you," he told me. "I didn't want a stepfather, I wanted a father. Why can't a boy have two fathers?" he asked with tears in his eyes.

I realized that my own fears from the past had limited my ability to give Aaron all of myself. I see many men hold themselves back because they are unsure of how much they should give. Aaron was telling me, "Don't be afraid. Give all you've got. I need you. I love you." We were both in tears as were the other men who were holding us in their loving embrace.

Manhood may be a difficult state to achieve, but it is not the "Big Impossible." It requires guidance and initiation. Most of all, it requires that we be open to change, be open to love, and be open to being the elders the young men and women of our communities desperately need.

Chapter 4

Male Menopause,
Not Me!
Overcoming Fear and Denial

When I began research for this book, I expected I would find major differences between what men and women go through at midlife. I initially pictured a chart showing menopause on one side and andropause on the other. I envisioned a neat separation, with women having one kind of "change of life," and men having a very different kind. We could each learn about the other, but the "otherness" seemed clear and distinct.

Yet, the more I delved into the physical, hormonal, psychological, social, and spiritual changes that men and women experience at midlife, the more similar they seemed. I concluded that while there are major differences, obviously, the similarities are quite overwhelming.

The first way to help men move through their denial is to recognize that male menopause (viropause or andropause) is as real and inevitable as adolescence or puberty.

I think of menopause as puberty in reverse. At puberty, our hormones are coming on line. During menopause, they are changing in the other direction. No one would doubt that both males and females go through puberty, even though it is only the females who begin their menstrual cycles.

It shouldn't surprise us to learn that there is a male counterpart to menopause, even though it is only the women who end their menstrual cycles. In a recent book, one author had some interesting things to say about this critical period of life:

Male menopause must be approached today with a different attitude, one that is self-valuing, rather than self-deprecating. Making the effort to change eating, smoking, sleeping, and exercise habits, or taking the time to experiment with hormone replacement or homeopathic practices to help rebalance the body around its new hormonal state, is not an issue of vanity, or attracting women, or succumbing to Western culture's preoccupation with youth. It is an issue of physical and mental health.

This book, then, has three purposes: First, to shatter the myths about male menopause. Second, to emphasize that male menopause is a health issue and to coach men in how to educate their doctors and the women in their lives. And finally, most important, I want to leave readers with another way to think about this stage of a man's life—what I call the Second Adulthood.

I found this book extremely helpful in focusing attention on the changes I was noticing as I approached fifty. The above quotes are accurate in every detail except one. In the original text, wherever the word "woman" appeared, I substituted "man," where it said "her" I wrote "him," where it said "menopause" I wrote "male menopause."

The quotes, in fact, are not from a book on male menopause, but from Gail Sheehy's *The Silent Passage: Menopause*. Yet, everything that she says about women, I believe applies to men.

Clearly the term "menopause" is not accurate as it applies to men. Men don't have a menstrual cycle and so they don't have an ending of a menstrual cycle. However, just as there is more to a woman's menopause than the moment she ovulates for the last time, there is much more to what men experience than a purely psychological midlife crisis. But this is often difficult for men to accept.

Our beliefs have such a strong influence on what we see in the world, they may blind us to the truth. I originally bought books on menopause to help me understand what my wife was going through. I have page after page underlined, with notes in the margin reading, "Exactly, right....That's what's happening to Carlin....That's her....She's going through the same thing." At the time, it never occurred to me that anything I read applied to me.

Since I "knew" menopause was something that all women went through and no men experienced, I never saw what was staring me in the face, that I was beginning to experience many of the symptoms that Carlin had gone through.

It reminds me of a story an anthropologist told of encountering natives who had been so isolated they had rarely seen a non-native person. Wanting to know what name they gave to various objects, he placed a number of things he carried in his pocket within a circle he had drawn on the ground. There was some change, a small knife, a cigarette, and a watch. The native man recognized and named all the objects he saw.

Yet, there was still one object left in the circle. The anthropologist kept prodding the man to name the last object. The native man insisted that he had already named everything, that there was nothing left in the circle to name. The anthropologist finally concluded that the man had never seen a watch before and therefore it didn't register as an object in his brain. For him, the circle was empty.

This story illustrates an important point that applies to male and female menopause. What we believe about these human experiences will determine whether or not it exists for us and what we may choose to do about it. A psychologist friend reverses the old phrase, "I'll believe it when I see it," and says, "I'll see it when I believe it."

We're Both Going through Menopause

After reading the article about male menopause in the newspaper, I can see that both my wife and I are going through this together. I'm fifty-one and she's forty-nine and the symptoms you mentioned could apply equally well to both of us: emotional ups and downs, irritability, loss of sexual desire, weight gain, memory loss, fatigue, loss of fun and joy in our lives. As soon as she began experiencing the symptoms, she went to a doctor in a town not far from us. Even though I know I need help, too, I haven't done anything about it. I guess I've been embarrassed to admit I am having problems. I keep thinking it's a sign of weakness. I already feel like I'm losing something vital in my life and to admit I'm going through male menopause makes me feel even less manly. But I know I need to do something. Your article made me feel that I'm not so alone and that it's not unmanly to seek help. Do you have any suggestions about who I could see?

Ed

Points of understanding:

• Without a concept for male menopause, no one sees that it exists. Now that we have a concept, much of what we have been seeing for years makes sense. With this new perspective, men can recognize the similarities between what women are going through and what men are experiencing. When men see the symptoms set out in front of them, they often recognize themselves.

• Even with this recognition, they are reluctant to seek help. It has taken women a long while to accept menopause as a normal part of life, not something to be hidden or denied. It will take men some time to accept their change as well.

• Until there were many health care professionals who specialized in menopause, women often were told, "It's all in your head," "There's nothing we can do," "You just have to get through it." Now we know there are many options available.

• The understanding of male menopause is decades behind our understanding of female menopause. But men need help now and are reaching out for support. Until more people in health care understand male menopause, men will have to undertake a lot of education.

A woman friend who has been a leader in the women's movement over the last thirty years told me that she might believe there was such a thing as male menopause when she saw men having hot flashes. The sudden rise in temperature that makes a woman want to open the car window on a freezing December evening is often seen as the marker for menopause, something that women share and that men don't experience.

The truth is there are women who never experience hot flashes and men who do. Here's an example from a stack of many letters I've received from men.

Hot Flash!

My name is Albert and I'm thirty-six years old. I feel like I am going through male menopause, though no one seems to take it seriously but me. I have feelings of being hot all day and at night I wake up with the sheets drenched, even when it's quite cool.

I feel it even more when I'm stressed, but even when I'm just sitting around, I touch my arms or legs and they're hot. I don't have a fever and I'm not sick. My doctor has checked me out and says that there is nothing wrong with me. When I asked about male menopause, he just shook his head. My wife and kids laugh at me. They say I'm crazy. Maybe I am. Can you help?

Albert

Points of understanding:

• Dr. Malcolm Carruthers, who has done extensive research on more than two thousand men going through male menopause, found that 50 percent experience night sweats.

• Carruthers also found that 25 percent of men experience hot flashes. Although not as common as the hot flashes women experience, they can be very uncomfortable and difficult for men.

• Many people have experienced the frustration and shame of knowing something is not right with them and being told by a doctor that "it's nothing." Many know what it's liked to be ridiculed and laughed at by family members that don't understand.

• It is vital for us to break down these barriers to understanding so that men can get the help they need and families can work together rather than being pulled apart by male menopause.

• It shouldn't really surprise us that both men and women experience many of the same symptoms, including hot flashes, since both have hormonal changes at this time of life. Since women's hormones drop more rapidly than a man's, their physical symptoms are often more pronounced. However, we all know women who go through menopause with few physical symptoms and we know men who experience severe changes.

I Just Don't Get It

I have just started reading your book, *Male Menopause*, and I really didn't need to go much past the introduction to recognize what my husband and I are presently experiencing.

My husband left me in July after nearly twenty-six years of marriage. We have one son, who is twenty. William is now forty-seven and I am forty-six. We grew up on the same block and I always thought we would grow old together, now I'm not so sure.

We built a wonderful life together. I helped him finish college after we were married and he has had a successful career. The marriage was good, not perfect, but good, up until about two years ago.

William began having problems holding an erection and after about eight months or so of being treated by a urologist, he began to take Viagra. It was a very stressful time for both of us. The Viagra worked and I thought things would get better, but it was only the beginning.

About a year ago, William began talking about a possible job promotion that would take us to the Los Angeles area. I was not very supportive at first. Los Angeles is not where I would choose to live.

This past Easter, he informed me that he was pretty sure he was going to get the job, but that he didn't think he wanted me to go with him. He told me he loved me, but wasn't in love with me anymore. It was as if someone hit me in the face with a brick and I never saw it coming.

He tells me he feels empty…that he has no passion for anything. He tells me that he has always been someone's son, someone's brother, someone's husband, someone's father, and that one day he woke up and didn't know who he was anymore. He tells me he is not in love with me anymore, but that he will always love me. He will not see me or our son. He has completely left his life. He has no communication with his mother or nine brothers and sisters. He has no communication with our friends.

This is all so unlike William. We had a wonderful little family and he now he acts as if we don't exist. I just don't get it. He's acting crazy.

This is not the romantic man who wrote me wonderful cards on special occasions, telling how much he loved our life, our family, me. This is not the man who every year sends me yellow roses on the anniversary of the day that we met. William was a strong man, a kind man, a decent man, and a hard worker…really he is a workaholic.

He was not the type of man to abandon his family. He just ran away. Everyone who knows us cannot believe this has happened.

The summer before last, I saw flashes of anger from him over the stupidest things, like parking spaces. I knew something was going on with him. I thought it was the sexual problem and job pressure. I wish I would have known that it was so much more.

Dorothy

Points of understanding:

• Like so many women who have said of so many men, "he just doesn't get it," Dorothy just can't get what William has been saying. He has always been someone in relation to someone else. Midlife is a time when men cry out to be themselves.

• Men often speak their pain through their behavior, not their words. His irritability and sexual difficulties were ways he was expressing his unhappiness.

• In one of my previous books I talked about the "wisdom of the penis." When men have become numb to their feelings, cut off from their bodies, sometimes it is left to the penis to tell the truth. It may be shouting, "I'm sick and tired of this old existence. I'm not going to get up for another round, even if I have to disappoint myself and you." It isn't surprising that giving a man Viagra is often not helpful. It may restore an erection, but it also quiets the truth that wants to be spoken. In the end the truth will come out, sometimes with explosive results.

• William speaks for many men and women who find they have been playing so many relationship roles they have lost their relationship with themselves.

• A job change, or other significant change, is often the trigger to look at more fundamental feelings that a man has about his life.

• When we lose connection with ourselves, we lose our power and passion. We often feel the only way to reclaim ourselves is to totally cut ourselves off from our old life. There are better ways, but when we are scared we often don't seek them out.

• A destructive break with the past is not necessary if we can recognize the early warning signs and learn to support each other in creating a new life that works for the man and the woman.

• This period of a man's life is complicated. Beware of the quick fix, whether it is a small pill that will make everything OK, a job change, or a move to a new city. What is required is good information, sensitive communication, caring support, a high degree of patience, and a willingness to keep trying when things are the most difficult.

More Alike Than Different

I hope by now you have expanded your beliefs to accept the idea that male menopause, like the watch in the native's circle, exists. I hope you have also recognized that there are many similarities between what women go through—both emotionally and physically—during menopause and what men go through.

Listening to Carlin's women's group discuss their experiences with menopause and listening to my own men's group go over the same territory, I was struck by how similar the issues were. If someone were reading the transcripts of the two groups and didn't know in advance which was the men's group and which was the women's group, their gender wouldn't be immediately obvious.

Contrary to the myth that men and women are from different planets, we are much more alike than different, and the differences we do see are greatest during the reproductive years. As we approach the menopause years, the changes that men and women experience can draw us together.

"There are many things women and men of middle age have in common," says Rosetta Reitz, author of *Menopause: A Positive Approach*, "and to know about the other is to learn more about oneself. A sympathetic viewing of female menopause would teach men a lot about their own." This is also true for women in viewing male menopause.

Trouble Reaching Out

We sometimes think of menopause as being an easy topic for women to discuss and male menopause as something of a taboo topic. Until recently, menopause was also something that was rarely discussed in the open. When Gail Sheehy appeared on *The Oprah Winfrey Show* in 1992 to discuss her new book, *The Silent Passage*, Oprah's producer admitted on the air that they had had an easier time booking guests to talk about murdering their spouses than about menopause. In the last eight to ten years, menopause has come into the mainstream and millions of women are getting the benefit of new approaches and treatments.

Men are still lagging behind women in this respect. Men just don't like to admit that they go through changes, particularly changes that go to the core of their sense of manhood. They also have a difficult time admitting to any problem they associate with something a woman has. The worst taunts a boy experienced growing up was that he was acting like a girl. If a girl was quiet, he had to be loud. If she was soft, he had to be hard. If she was gentle, he had to be tough. If she was emotional, he was unemotional. If she went through menopause, he…well he didn't have hormonal cycles or physiological changes. He stayed forever young, or did his best to deny any problems associated with aging.

A fifty-six-year-old therapist came into our health clinic the other day. He seemed angry, looked at his watch, and was obviously wanting to get out as soon as possible. I had heard about Marty over the years from his wife who came in for regular checkups, but I had never seen him before. Even before I could ask him why he was visiting me, he burst forth. "My wife made the appointment for me and said she'd leave me if I didn't keep it," he grumbled. "I know what you're going to tell me. I need to lower my cholesterol, stop smoking, cut down on my drinking, and eat better. I don't need a so-called expert to tell me that. I just need to do it on my own."

I see many men like Marty. In general, women are much more likely to seek help and support for anything, including health-related issues. Why? Perhaps it's as Andrew Kimbrell, a cofounder of the Men's Health Network, suggests: "In their twenties, men are too strong to see a doctor. In their thirties, they're too busy, and in their forties, they're too scared they might have a disease they neglected to pay attention to in their twenties and thirties."

A recent survey showed how reticent men are to reach out for help. Most of the fifteen hundred physicians surveyed agreed that, compared with women, men:

• have more trouble discussing health concerns, particularly concerns about sexuality or hormones.

• are less likely to seek medical attention for a health complaint.

• are more likely to delay treatment for a known problem until their condition worsens.

• are less likely to stick with a treatment plan.

If men are reluctant to discuss such things as cholesterol, smoking, drinking, and eating, think how much more reluctant they are to talk about issues of virility, vitality, sexuality, intimacy, life goals, and aging. All these issues, and many others, are part of male menopause and require our attention.

So, how do we get through to men? How do we help men who don't believe they are going through male menopause? How do we educate a predominantly male medical establishment to the realities of male menopause? It isn't easy, but it can be done.

Overcoming Male Denial: Helping Men Who Don't Know They Need Help

The question I am asked over and over is, "How can I get through to a man who doesn't realize he is going through male menopause or isn't willing to receive help?" It isn't always easy, but there are ways I have found that work.

1. Start with You

As a therapist who has been working with individuals and couples over the last thirty-five years, I often have half of the couple coming in wanting "help" for the other person. Often, the woman is trying to get her husband to change something so their relationship will improve. She's hoping for some magic wisdom I can give her that will transform her husband and help him lead a more joyful and productive life. The first question I ask is, "How would your life be better if he changed?"

When I asked that question of Dora, a forty-six-year-old woman who was concerned about her husband's menopausal symptoms, she was at first taken aback. "Well, I never thought of it in terms of *my* life. I just wanted him to get better." When she thought more about it, things began to focus on Dora's needs. "I feel like I'm losing the man I love," she said as tears began to flow. "He's become distant and withdrawn and I'm afraid he'll either leave or stay, but remain withdrawn from me."

You can't help another person while you are so out of balance or so much in pain that your own survival depends on the other person changing. It puts too much pressure on the relationship. You have to start with you. I began to get Dora to think about what she could do to feel better, whether her husband, Henry, was ready to change or not. She began to spend more time with friends and family, worked out regularly at the local gym, and changed the way she was eating.

Men are much more likely to look at their own situation when they are seeing the woman in their life doing good things for herself, rather than trying to get him to change.

My Husband Won't Do Anything to Help Himself

I am going through the devastation of my husband's midlife. It has been a living hell. Some men will talk about what they're going through, be willing to seek some help, or at least admit, even to themselves, something is wrong. My husband won't. He says he has no problems. He refuses to read anything. He won't go to counseling. He won't take the Zoloft medicine he was prescribed. It made a tremendous difference for the six weeks he took it and he didn't know he was taking it for depression. He didn't seek this help, I went to our doctor and he worked with me.

I have been going to counseling. My doctor there said she believes my husband needs help to get through this.

Maybe it is hopeless, but I can't seem to let it go. I still love him. As difficult, devastating, and emotionally draining as this all is, I don't want to give up. But I can't keep doing this forever. It is tearing me apart. He is stuck right now and I feel in limbo. He doesn't see the path of destruction he is leaving behind him. Have you ever tried to explain to an adorable two-year-old granddaughter as she looks into your eyes at her birthday party and says, "Where's grandpa?" that his problems are keeping him away from her? They had an incredibly close relationship before male menopause hit.

We have been happily married for twenty-five years. If this condition truly has men believing they feel this way, how can they ever be helped?

Joyce

Points of understanding:

• Often, the first step in helping him is to help yourself. There are many ways to help a man move past his resistance and denial.

• Sometimes a man needs some "hard love" to wake him up to the loss of family that his behavior is costing. At other times he needs gentle understanding.

• I've seen the most hopeless situations turn around. The key is to take care of yourself so you don't destroy yourself trying to save him.

2. Learn All You Can about Male and Female Menopause

Read, talk to friends, get information. Don't make this so much about him. Make it more about you learning about this very interesting and complex life transition. Although this is a difficult transition for many, the good news is that it means you have made it this far in life. Remember, for most people, through most of human history, menopause was not something they worried about. When death came at forty or forty-five, they didn't get a chance to experience the next phase of adulthood or the menopause transition that leads to it.

The purpose of menopause, male and female, is to prepare us for the next phase of our adult lives, which can be the most powerful, passionate, and productive we have yet experienced. It can be a time of emotional and spiritual growth, a time when old wounds are finally healed, a time when we don't have to strive so hard for success but can enjoy the life we are given, a time of self-acceptance and gratitude, and a time of gift giving for the generations who follow us.

3. Share Your Information

Men learn more about male menopause from women than they do from other men. Most of the early research on male menopause was conducted by women health care professionals who were studying menopause and began to wonder whether there were similar changes going on with men. As they shared their knowledge, more and more people began to recognize that male menopause was a real phenomenon and that it did similar things to men as menopause did to women.

As women learn more about male menopause, they are educating their doctors, their women and men friends, as well as their husbands. I've gotten hundreds of letters from men who said they first heard about male menopause when a woman gave them a copy of the "Dear Abby" article or a copy of my book.

The key to educating men is to offer information without the expectation that he change. If he doesn't feel pushed, he's more likely to get past his denial. "I never would have written you this letter," said Zachary, "if my wife hadn't shown me the article in our local newspaper. It was pretty clear from the list of symptoms that I'm going through male menopause."

"I found your book sitting on my bedstand a month ago," wrote Jake. "I laughed, thought it was some kind of joke and put it back on my wife's side of the bed. It kept appearing on my side. She never said a word. I just kept seeing the book. I finally opened it and found pages starred and sections underlined. I read a few, never thinking any of it could apply to me, but there I was. I felt like you had been looking in on my life. Thanks."

"I knew he needed to read the book as soon as I saw it, but I also knew that any effort on my part to interest him would cause him to run the other direction," Marjorie wrote. "I decided to make the book so mysterious and attractive he would want to read it on his own. I put a book cover over it so he couldn't see the title and took it with me wherever I went. When he asked what I was reading, I told him, 'just a book,' and wouldn't give him any details. I would read by myself and often make exclamations, 'Wow…that's amazing!' I didn't have to fake it. I was really into it. 'What?' he would ask me. 'I know you wouldn't be interested,' I'd reply. I left it behind one day and when I came home he was sitting reading it. He tried to hide it at first, but then admitted that the suspense was driving him crazy and after reading a few chapters he admitted it was actually pretty interesting."

There are many ways of sharing the information. Some men will respond with the direct approach, others need to find the truth themselves (with a little help from their friends).

4. Recognize That Many People See Menopause, Particularly Male Menopause, As the Beginning of the End

If menopause is the transition to this most wonderful time of life, why do so many people avoid it like the plague? One woman described her fears this way. "I remember my mother going through menopause and it seemed that life was all downhill from there. Her hot flashes seemed to permanently burn her insides. She become all dried up, lost interest in life, and wanted to be left alone. I saw what it did to my father. He lost the woman he loved and he grew more morose and withdrawn as the years went on. They definitely didn't have a happy old age.

"Although I've read enough and talked to enough friends to know I don't have to follow in my mother's footsteps, I'm still afraid it will happen to me. I can't see anything wonderful in getting old. If there is a post-menopausal zest, I'm not sure I'll have any."

As we learn more about menopause and aging, women are beginning see that this period of life can be positive. It is still difficult for men.

I Feel Like I'm Fading Away

I am a forty-six-year-old man and feel I am in the midst of what you call male menopause. I lack energy, sexual drive, and feel depressed. I feel there is something "great" I need to do, but feel it's really too late to do it, even if I knew what it was. I recently had an affair, which made me feel young again, but it didn't last long. I came back to my wife feeling guilty and ashamed.

I don't even know why I did it. When my wife was going through menopause, it nearly drove us apart. But I hung in there with her and we came back together. I felt our relationship was even stronger. But this seems different. I feel so old and worthless, even though I know, intellectually, I have a lot of good years ahead of me.

I feel like I am fading away, becoming less and less of a man as time goes on. I walk slower. I have lost the bounce in my step. My self-esteem is extremely fragile. The slightest thing can plunge me into a depressed mood.

I've become afraid of having sex with my wife. I think constantly about losing my erection. I bring our new puppy into bed with us so I don't have to face the fear.

I hate my job—no, I don't really hate it. I just feel I've outgrown it. I'd like to start over with a new career, but I know I'm too old.

Points of understanding:

• That feeling of being old is not just something that we imagine. We do live in a youth-oriented culture that still sees younger as better and older as bad.

A recent segment of CBS's *Sixty Minutes* TV documentary described the meteoric fall of a teenage prodigy—screenwriter and actress Riley Weston—whose career ended abruptly when the entertainment industry learned that her true age was thirty-two.

Once hailed as a "nineteen-year-old who could write for nineteen-year-olds," Weston had a contract with Disney to develop her own series and a dazzling future before her. Yet, when the "bombshell" news of her age hit the wires, her phone stopped ringing immediately.

But age bias is not only present in the entertainment industry, it is pervasive everywhere. According to Nina Munk, whose article "Finished at Forty" appeared in the February 1999 issue of *Fortune* magazine, "In America, basketball players, dancers, and fashion models are finished young. Mathematicians and chess players peak early, too.

"Once you're fifty-five," she continues, "it's almost impossible to find a job in business. But a new trend is emerging: in corporate America, forty is starting to look and feel old." As more and more companies "downsize" to save money, they terminate large numbers of older workers, rather than those most recently hired, when they reduce the size of their workforce.

For men who base a great deal of their identity and feelings of manhood on their ability to work and be productive, even the thought that they may not be able to find work is terrifying.

5. Don't Try and Cheer Him Up, Listen to His Feelings of Despair

When a man feels down, nothing fails more than trying to cheer him up by telling him, "Don't worry, everything will work out OK. Getting old isn't so bad. Things will get better." Before things can get better a man needs to be able to admit to someone he loves how awful he feels. Both men and women often collude in keeping him silent. He often will say, "I don't want to worry her with my problems." She often will admit, "Though I do want him to open up to me, I'm afraid my big strong man will fall apart. I'm so used to him handling any crisis without complaint, I have trouble accepting his fear and weakness."

One of the greatest gifts one person can give to another is to listen openly and feel with them without trying to change the other person. The message is, "I'm with you no matter what. We'll get through whatever we might face together."

6. Move Beyond Despair to Risk Loving Communication

Until a person can accept how he really feels, there is little room to move ahead. As long as he denies what is truly going on inside him, he will remain stuck. The best way to heal is to recognize the issues and work to discuss them openly. Most people, particularly men, when faced with difficulties, want to immediately move to solve the problem. But sometimes, there is no silver bullet. Open communication between a couple may take time, but it is the best way to move toward understanding.

She Let Me Know She Cared

I felt like everything in my life was falling apart. It seemed that whatever I did, I made things worse. My wife and I were fighting all the time. Even though I'd swear after each fight that I'd never let it happen again, a month, a week, a day, or even an hour later, she would say something that would trigger me and we'd start all over again.

I would escape into my work, but it didn't really help. A creeping feeling of hopelessness began to envelope me like a fog. I felt I was suffocating. I wanted to scream for help, but I knew no one would understand. I was totally alone.

One night after I had worked late and gone out for a few drinks, I came home expecting my wife to jump on me for being late. Instead, she took me by the hand and we sat together on the couch. She had a fire going in the fireplace. I felt suspicious at first, but her touch was soft. The first words out of her mouth melted the ice that had encrusted my heart. "I love you, Jason. I don't want to lose you. I know you've been going through hell inside. I'm here, no matter what. Do you want to talk to me?" Her voice was so kind and gentle, it pierced through my defenses.

I was so choked up, no words came out at first, but soon they began to pour out. I couldn't believe she really wanted to hear it all—the frustration, the anger, the despair, the thoughts of leaving, the fears of suicide. I wanted to protect her, but I kept letting it out. She just kept holding my hand and telling me, "Keep going, I'm here."

That evening didn't solve all our problems, not by any means, but it started us on a path. I could begin to recognize the changes I was going through. I could stop blaming her and stop blaming myself. I began reading about male menopause and began to see myself in the stories of others. I began to come out of the fog for the first time in many years. Now, three years into the process, I can see some light at the end of the tunnel.

That one night when Linda really allowed me to let it out, let me know she cared about me and about us, and let me know she would stick with me, made all the difference in the world. I guess I was convinced that if I really let out all the shit I was carrying inside, no one would really want to stay with me. Or if they did want to stay, it would be only out of pity, not out of love.

I know I have a lot of work to do, but now I know I'm not alone. I've even begun to talk to some of my male friends and find many of them are going through the same kind of changes. We are actually talking about male menopause and what we can do to get through this.

7. You Can Help Him See That Many of His Problems Have a Common Root

Peter was fifty-five when he came to see me. He said he had been having one problem after another but couldn't get a handle on what was going on. He began having prostate problems in his forties and had seen a urologist who prescribed antibiotics and later told him he had an enlarged prostate and gave him medications for that. When he hit fifty, he began to have problems keeping an erection. "That really scared me," he said. "I denied there was anything happening for two or three years, but finally went to see my doctor who prescribed Viagra.

"I've been feeling fatigued for years and tried everything under the sun, but no one has found the cause.

"Last year, I got injured playing football on the weekend and I can't jog or do much exercising, which makes me feel depressed. I've seen a psychiatrist to treat the depression which he feels I've had for a long time.

"Even my relationship seems to be in trouble. We don't fight, but we don't communicate well, either. We seem to live in separate worlds. I feel like the little Dutch boy who sticks his finger in the dike, only to find a new leak coming through. I'm running out of fingers and toes to stop the flow and I'm worried that it will break through soon."

Some men have come to recognize there is a problem, but don't see the big picture. They don't see that all the symptoms are part of a larger whole. Part of the problem is our current view of health care that treats each separate part rather than the whole. Another is our lack of understanding of male menopause even within the health care community. A specialist versed in every symptom of male menopause could help men and their families see the whole picture. At my clinic, I treat male menopause as a hormonal, physical, psychological, interpersonal, sexual, social, and spiritual change of life.

What you can do is help him see the "forest," not just the "trees." Sometimes its as simple as showing him my article from the Dear Abby column or leaving information on the subject where he can find it, or sharing your own experience of the change of life.

He's Tried It All

I am reading your book, *Male Menopause*. I currently have nineteen doctors, four of whom are psychiatrists. I have been through every department except the morgue. I am on twenty-three different medications, from Atarax to Viagra to Zantac—most of the time I'm in a stupor. I'm fifty-two years old this month and after four years of different medications and doctors, I see little improvement. Of course, I had to take medical leave from being VP of a large advertising company. Essentially, I am being treated for obsessive compulsive disorder (OCD), anxiety, and severe depression.

I should add that as a child from the ages of four to thirteen I was sexually molested by an uncle. I thought I had gotten rid of this unwanted baggage until five years ago it came to the forefront. I find that I have every symptom you mention. The worst being these extreme hot flashes. I also have osteoporosis and testosterone levels that are low to borderline-low.

Last week, I brought your book and a few others on men's health to four different doctor's appointments and, much to my surprise, was almost laughed out of the place with a there's-no-such-thing attitude. I just cannot believe that they all were so closed-minded and ignorant about this subject. The time and money I and my insurance company have wasted is astronomical.

George

Points of understanding:

• This is an extreme example of what happens when a person is not diagnosed properly or offered the correct treatment. It also shows how difficult it is for even respected medical centers to understand the complex changes going on at this time of life.

• Male menopause can't be understood or treated with a purely medical approach. There is a need to treat the whole person, not just his symptoms. For that, the best approach is either a practitioner (very rare) who has experience in medicine, men's health, hormonal and physical changes at midlife, psychology of men's life changes through time, male depression and related disorders, male sexuality, and spirituality, or a multidisciplinary team (also rare) of practitioners who can focus on the whole man and his changes.

• It is very common for long-buried trauma's from the past, such as child abuse, to surface. This can be very uncomfortable to deal with, but also can be the opportunity to heal past wounds that were buried but still cause problems.

• Although we think of hot flashes and osteoporosis as ailments that beset women as they get older, men also have these problems and need attention if they are to be fully functional as they age. Although conventional medical wisdom, at least in the United States, hasn't reached this level of understanding, more and more evidence suggests that replacing men's testosterone as it declines can protect men from a variety of age-related conditions, including heart disease and prostate problems, as well as osteoporosis and hot flashes.

8. You Can Help Him See That This Is Not Something He Can Get through Alone

Most men are trained from childhood to be independent rather than interdependent. Even when they recognize they have a problem, they want to take care of it themselves. "No one can help me change, but me," Roger told me in his booming voice. He had agreed to see me for one session to satisfy his wife. "Look, don't get me wrong, I know I've got some things I need to work on, but I've got to do it myself. No offense, Doc, but I don't need anyone telling me how to make things better in my life. I can handle it."

Roger, like most men, grew up with images of *The Lone Ranger* and all the cowboys and heroes that taught us that real men take care of business themselves. Asking for help is for sissies and cry-babies and most men would rather die than risk being seen that way. Helping him break through his isolation isn't easy, but it's well worth the effort.

How Can I Support Him without Being Pushy?

My husband is fifty-three and suffers from nearly every symptom you mentioned. He has suffered from most of the emotional disorders you mentioned and many of the physical ones: depression, feelings of "invisibility" and lack of self-esteem, irritability, headaches, backaches, sleep disorders, intimacy problems, and more.

We are desperate for help, but no one here seems to take the problem seriously. Perhaps even more importantly, though, my husband recognized himself in the column and acknowledged that your letter hit the nail on the head for him. But he chooses not to seek help, thinking sometimes that he is not worth it or that nothing works, and other times that he can fix it by himself or that he shouldn't need someone else or medications or whatever to help him get well.

He did seek counseling at one time for depression and was on Prozac for two months, but he did not return to the prescribing psychiatrist, saying he felt much better and didn't think he needed any more treatment. He did improve on Prozac (I saw this, and told him so), but he now believes it made no difference and has pretty much closed the door to further medications.

How can I be supportive without being pushy?
Clara

Fortunately, men are breaking free of this destructive life pattern. They are recognizing that being a man does not have to mean suffering in silence. Sometimes it's hard for a woman to get through to a resistant man without being pushy and creating more resistance. This is the place where other men can be particularly helpful. Men at midlife often feel the need to have more contact with men. Some reach out to other men who share in business, others reach out through the Rotary, Elks, and other traditional men's organizations, still others reach out to men in the gym where they work out, and some join men's groups for mutual support.

In various ways, men can begin to support each other's health and move from an ideal of isolated independence to interdependence.

Most men aren't likely to respond well if a woman tells him, "I think you are too isolated, why don't you join a men's group." However, if she encourages any move in that direction he does make, he is more likely to take another step. Many men I know get involved in a men's group after their wives join a women's group. When he sees how much support she gets, he may be less likely to sit home alone when she is out and instead reach out to other men.

As men make more connections with other men at this time of life, openings begin to happen that allow them to talk more personally about life changes and get support for recognizing that male menopause is something we all go through. Going through it with other men can make the journey less difficult and more joyful.

9. You Can Help Him See That the Quick Fix Won't Work

We are a quick-fix society. We want our help to be fast, simple, and easy. "Give me the pill that will take off the pounds," she says. "I want the pill that will give me the sexual stamina of a twenty-year-old," he tells me.

I've talked with many men who begin to get help, but then stop before real change can occur. They often try the quick fix over and over before they recognize that health sometimes comes faster if we go more slowly and take our time.

"I knew I was going through male menopause when I read your article," said George, "But I wanted things fixed quickly. I was too busy with life to slow down long enough to see what was really going on." George was here for the second time. I had seen him a year previously, but he dropped out of counseling after a few sessions. "I didn't even want to take time for a complete physical," he recalled. "When you tried to explain the importance of getting a full picture of me and my life before we decided what to do, I didn't want to hear it. I just wanted Viagra and was sure it would solve all my problems. I went to another doctor who was happy to give me the prescription I wanted.

"Not only didn't it solve things, I think it actually made things worse for my wife and I. I thought if I got my sexual desire back and could keep an erection, everything would fall into place. Joyce wasn't ready to just jump into bed again. She said we needed to build back our relationship, to learn to be partners again. I guess she's right, but why does it have to be so complicated?"

Sticking with your desire to have a full and satisfying relationship, not settling for a quick fix that doesn't really fix anything, helps give him the patience and courage to go the distance.

Moving through male menopause takes years. There is no quick way to get through it. However, *slow* and *easy* will get you there a lot sooner than *fast* and *furious*.

10. You Can Help Him Stick with a Program When He's Given Up

Raymond came in for help after reading my book. "I can see myself in almost every page," he began. "All these years I thought I was just getting old and falling apart. I didn't know there was something I could actually do."

We treated Raymond's depression with a combination of antidepressants, exercise, and cognitive-behavior therapy. We helped him change his eating habits so he could lose weight and feel more physically fit. We treated his testosterone deficiency with a replacement program that helped restore his strength, vigor, and sexual desire.

We worked with him on his relationship and helped him look at what he wanted to do with his life after he retired. After two years at the clinic, he seemed well on his way to achieving his goals and reclaiming the life that had seemed to be going downhill. Just when things were going well, he stopped coming.

According to his wife, Janine, "He told me everything is fine now. I don't need medications, I'm done with counseling, I can handle things on my own now. And things did go well, for a time. Then the dark moods came back and he began drinking more heavily again. He says he's considering coming back, but hasn't decided yet."

In the clinic I am associated with, we want people to be on their own as soon as they can, but not to leave too soon and revert back to destructive behavior. The way I handle this is to encourage regular check-ins after a person leaves. I tell them it is like dental hygiene. If you only see the dentist in a crisis, you lose the opportunity to detect problems early on.

We found if we build in opportunities for regular checkups, the man doesn't feel like he's failed if problems begin to reoccur or to feel ashamed for leaving the clinic.

What a partner can do is to keep the vision. Janine didn't leave counseling just because Raymond felt he no longer needed help. She kept regular checkups going, so that when Raymond was ready for additional support, the line of communication was already open.

What Do You Do When You've Tried These Steps and You Still Can't Get through to Him?

When a man opens up and his feelings pour out, it is like nothing else in the world. Many women tell me, "I never knew there was so much pain inside him." Men tell me, "I never knew I had so much bottled up inside." For both it is a new beginning that makes all the work worthwhile.

I am convinced that this reconnection is possible for everyone. I have seen the most destructive relationships find renewal and rebirth with the right support. I have seen the most closed and resistant men open their hearts when given the right nutrients of love. Sometimes, however, things don't work out. There is too much pain, too many layers of armor built up.

So, let's deal with the worst case first. I tell my clients if they can deal with the thing they fear the most, it will help free them from that fear and move ahead with their lives.

You Can End the Relationship

For many, ending the relationship is something they fear more than anything. They say, "I love him, I just can't give up on us." They have done everything they know how to do and being in the relationship has become self-destructive. The fighting may have become so severe that there is physical violence involved. Or, things may have settled into a cold war which causes violence to our heart and soul. Even our physical selves can become sick under these circumstances. Many people faced with a relationship that is killing them and a belief that they can't leave become physically ill. They may even develop heart disease, cancer, or some other life-threatening ailment.

Some people will stay on a sinking ship and die rather than jump overboard and take a chance of saving their lives. One of the first questions I ask a person in these circumstances is, "If things didn't get better and you felt you were going under, would you be willing to leave?" For some, that is the most difficult decision of their lives.

JoAnne was one of those people. She had been married to David for thirty years. They had met in high school, knew they were right for each other from the very beginning, and were sure they would raise a family and spend their whole lives together. "When David began having problems, I was totally confused. He became withdrawn and angry. I did everything I knew to be helpful. I got him to go to his doctor, we changed our diets, we took a stress-reduction class. Things would improve for awhile, but would slip back into the same old patterns. He finally stopped listening to me. I knew he was discouraged, but I couldn't reach him. He shut me out.

"Over the years, we just went along, doing our work and living in the same house. I knew I was dying inside, but I couldn't give up.

I got books, I went to therapy. I felt better, but I couldn't, I wouldn't give up on David. I knew we were both slowly dying, but I couldn't let go." JoAnne burst into tears.

The first thing I had to teach JoAnne was that leaving was not giving up. In fact, it was just the opposite. If she stayed, it was clear that both she and David would continue to go downhill until one or both of them was emotionally or physically dead. Leaving was life-affirming. I helped her say to David, "I love myself too much to die for your disease. I love you too much to sit quietly and watch you die." Leaving may turn out to be the end of the relationship or it can be the catalyst that brings it back to life.

You Can Leave the Relationship and Let It Breathe

This is what JoAnne did. She finally moved out, got her own apartment, and reestablished her own life. "I realized I had been keeping a death watch for years waiting for David to come to his senses, but believing that nothing would really change. I didn't know how dead I felt until I left. I was suffocating, but wasn't aware that the air was getting stale. It happened so slowly, I didn't see what was happening.

"It was the hardest decision I have ever made. But I know it was the right thing. I wasn't doing David any good to die with him. I want to live with him and regain the life we once had, or create a new one that is even better.

"I was sure David would just drift away. He didn't seem to have any interest in the relationship while we were together, so it surprised me when he called and wanted to get together for coffee. I'm not sure where things will go from here, but I know I'll never go back to a relationship that is killing us."

I've worked with many couples like JoAnne and David. Sometimes it takes a crisis to shake things up enough to make a major change. It took JoAnne's leaving to break through David's resistance. The first thing he came to realize was that he didn't want to lose her and was willing to come in for counseling to see if their relationship could be saved.

Sometimes leaving a relationship is the only way to breathe new life into it. Sometimes leaving a man is the only way to get him know what he could lose. Either way, it takes a willingness to risk everything, to put it all on the line. There are times this is necessary, but it is good if a couple can deal with male menopause before this stage.

You Can Resist the Temptation to See Yourself As the Problem

For many men, male menopause is the most frustrating and confusing time of life that they ever have experienced. Most men are action-oriented and look outside themselves to solve problems. When midlife brings changes, they often look elsewhere for understanding.

Rafael was a typical fifty-four-year-old man who was convinced that the life changes he was experiencing were caused by others. The list of others that were making his life miserable went on and on:

• "The children never write or call, and when they do they always want to talk to their mother. They only care about me when they want money."

• "I'm not appreciated at work. The younger guys get the raises and I don't get any respect."

• "The country is going to hell in a handbasket. All the politicians are a bunch of crooks who give themselves raises while spending our money."

• "Everyone wants something. Women want more, minorities want more, the poor want more. How about us working slobs? What do we get? Not a damn thing!"

All the frustrations that Rafael was feeling seemed to be focused like a laser beam on his wife, Barbara. "He used to be so caring and considerate. He never forgot a birthday or anniversary, bought me flowers 'just because,' and was romantic in so many special ways. But over the last few years, it seems like I've become his enemy. The more I try and please him, the more he complains.

"Sometimes he gets so angry, even over the smallest things, I'm afraid he is going to hit me. At times, he's broken things in the house, thrown an ashtray across the room which almost hit me, and smashed his fist into the wall.

"He tells me I've become a lousy housekeeper, that I've put on too much weight, that I spend too much money, that I talk on the phone all the time. Sometimes I feel he has a right to be angry. I *have* let myself go a bit and I do spend money, but never extravagantly. If I didn't talk on the phone I think I'd go crazy. He's suspicious of everything I do these days and quizzes me when I come back. What can I do to make him see that the problem isn't all me?"

The first thing I helped Barbara recognize is that she couldn't "make him" do anything. The key to breaking the old pattern was for her to learn to set better boundaries about what kind of behavior she would tolerate. I helped her see that her first commitment was to be sure she was safe. I coached her on talking to Rafael at times when they were calm. "Look Rafael, I love you and I know you love me. It just isn't acceptable for us to get to a place where you scream at me and throw things. It scares me too much. If it happens again, I want you to know that I'll leave the house immediately and stay with a friend. I'll come back in a few hours when things cool off between us."

She wasn't asking Rafael to change. Barbara was setting a clear boundary, one based on love for herself and for Rafael. She let him know that she'd be back, that she wasn't running out on him, just taking a break until things settled down.

Since Rafael could no longer vent his frustrations on Barbara, little by little he began to see that something was going on inside him. As Barbara continued to express her love and support, but was unwilling to be blamed for his unhappiness, he began to open up to his own pain. It can take a long time for this process to change from blame to acceptance of responsibility. Sometimes therapy is necessary for one or both partners, but change is possible.

He Became Obsessed with a Woman at Work

My husband, who will turn fifty next year, became obsessed with a twenty-nine-year-old at his workplace and is now living with her. Our two children and I are trying desperately to heal from this betrayal, but at the same time we are trying to understand why it happened. My husband had been a faithful, loving, and dedicated husband up until about a year ago. At that time, he began to worry about growing old and was concerned about getting gray hair, a paunchy tummy, etc.

I did all I could to assure him that he was as attractive as ever. However, this young woman was very aggressive and had a history of affairs with married men. I even gave him a second chance when I found out, and although he tried for awhile, he was unable to stay away from her.

I deal daily with feelings of guilt, dwelling on what I could have done to help prevent this. I am amazed at the number of couples we know who have gone through similar situations once they reach twenty to thirty years of marriage. My twenty-one-year-old daughter is also tormented by this crisis and is eager to learn more.

Dee

Points of understanding:

• When men ignore the warning signs of male menopause, it can lead to obsessions, misplaced affections, and even to addictions to alcohol and drugs.

• Although we often focus on the midlife male's attraction to younger women, younger women are often attracted to midlife men. They often are drawn to the status and power older men have achieved, or they are trying to find the love they never received from their fathers. Often, a wife is helpless to warn her husband of the danger. She, after all, has a vested interest in him staying. Men need their male friends to point out to them when they are acting inappropriately or getting involved in relationships that could be harmful to themselves and their families.

• We are just beginning to focus our attention on male menopause. No one should feel guilty that we haven't understood sooner what a man goes through at this time of life. Everyone did the best they could, knowing what they knew at the time.

• Learn what you can now, take care of yourself, and let him know that you love him and want your marriage to change and grow so both your needs and his needs can be met.

15 Things You Can Do to Help Once Male Menopause Is Recognized

All men are different and there is no formula that works for everyone. However there are a number of things that can helpful.

1. Recognize the similarities and differences between male and female menopause. The better informed you are, the more you'll be able to give helpful information.

2. Have patience, don't give up when things become difficult.

3. Be gentle and kind with yourself and your man.

4. Recognize that this is probably the most difficult and confusing time of life for both of you.

5. Take good care of yourself. Attend to your own needs and be sure you feel good on all seven levels—hormonally, physically, emotionally, interpersonally, sexually, socially, and spiritually.

6. Accept that he likely will be resistant at first to the concept of male menopause. Take your time in helping him move through his fear at his own pace.

7. He likely will be concerned, at first, with one or two aspects of male menopause. For instance, he may express concerns with physical or emotional aspects.

8. Listen to his concerns. It's tempting to want to get him to *do* something. Remember the first step to action is acknowledging there is a problem.

9. Keep listening. He may complain a lot about problems before he is ready to do something about them.

10. Reassure him that you love him and the two of you will get through this together.

11. Let him know that, though you understand this is a difficult time for him, you will not stand by and allow yourself to be abused by his words or actions.

12. Seek support together. Books can be useful tools for opening communication on the subject.

13. Many men are resistant to taking advice from a woman, particularly when the men are vulnerable and afraid. Sometimes getting another man—a friend or colleague—involved can be helpful.

14. Talk to him about what you see and feel. Particularly emphasize the positive things that can be done during this time of life.

15. Seek professional counseling if things remain stuck. Sometimes this period is so difficult that old behaviors and beliefs get locked in. Counseling can help open things up so that healthy change can begin to occur.

8 Things You Should Not Do

1. Don't ignore the changes that occur at this time of life. Male menopause is as natural as puberty and as impossible to ignore.

2. Don't panic. Your wonderful man has not turned into a monster, though like his adolescent counterpart, it may seem like he has.

3. Don't blame yourself. Many women are sure they must have done something wrong, particularly when a man begins to blame the woman for his own problems.

4. Don't be afraid to talk to others. Seek out your friends, your clergy, your doctor.

5. Don't laugh at your man or ridicule his behavior, even to your friends. Men's greatest fear at this stage of their lives is that they are acting like fools. Love and support him, even if his behavior is hard to take.

6. Don't let him make you the brunt of his anger. Men often act out at this stage and blame those close to them for their pain.

7. Don't give up on yourself, on him, or on the relationship. If it's worth keeping, it's worth fighting for.

8. Don't try too hard to make his life better. Ultimately, this is his change of life and he must navigate it for himself.

Chapter 5

———

Helping Your Man Move through the Seven Doorways of Male Menopause

"In the case of male menopause, we are still in the Dark Ages. Men have fewer guideposts to help them today than women had a generation ago. Only recently have we begun to understand the bio-chemistry of these events, tilting the scales toward a physiological explanation." — Theresa L. Crenshaw, M.D., author of *The Alchemy of Love and Lust.*

Now that a man is open to the possibility that he is going through male menopause, what can he do to successfully move through it? I picture this as a man coming down the Mountain of First Adulthood. Male menopause is what he experiences coming down this mountain and moving through the valley on his way to the Mountain of Second Adulthood. Though it may be uncomfortable, it is absolutely necessary. We can't move ahead in our lives unless we are willing to let go of the old baggage.

This is frightening for most of us, since it was our old baggage we relied on for our entire lives up until now. We may understand the concept that the old ways no longer work, that there is a new "us" waiting to emerge. But when it's late at night and we haven't been able to sleep, when our joints ache and our worries rise, when our relationship is in flux and our job is in jeopardy, when our sex life seems to be going the way of the dodo bird and our future seems as bright as dirt, it's not easy to see that there is something much better ahead of us.

We need to break through our denial to see the possibilities for the future and when we see a more hopeful future, it is easier to break through our denial.

There are those who accept that male menopause is real, but believe it simply has to do with a reduction of testosterone. The treatment of choice is simple—testosterone replacement therapy. I believe that male menopause is much more complex and a much more interesting stage of life. In fact, there are seven dimensions to male menopause and we must attend to them all if we are to treat the whole man.

At the Third Age Wellness Center, we deal with all aspects of a man's life. We think of the journey at this time of life as moving through seven doorways. We've heard from a lot of men and women who have sought help. Let's take a closer look at the new opportunities available for men as they deal with these areas of change in their lives.

Doorway #1: The Hormonal Symphony of Men: Keeping It in Tune

The endocrine system, which is composed of the cells and tissues that produce hormones, plays a key role in the male menopause process. A hormone is a substance produced in the body, usually in a gland, that is secreted into the bloodstream, travels through the body, and exerts its effects on some other gland or tissue of the body. The profound effects that hormones have on virtually all cells of the body, and the fact that the level of several hormones falls with age, explain why hormone replacement therapy has often been touted as a means of staying healthy as we age.

For women at midlife, emphasis has often been placed on hormonal shifts while psycho-social changes have been neglected. For men the reverse has been true. The psychological and social aspects of the male "midlife crisis" have been emphasized and less attention has been focused on male hormonal rhythms.

"It is safe to say that most physicians today do not believe male midlife crisis has a physical basis," says Dr. Crenshaw, "and treat it with psychotherapy and antidepressant medication—the same approach they used for female menopause decades ago."

Although testosterone replacement therapy has not been adopted by mainstream medicine in the U.S., this is beginning to change.

"Various studies on men with low testosterone levels have confirmed that testosterone replacement restores sex drive, erection, orgasm, ejaculation, and nocturnal erections," Dr. Crenshaw reports. "The biggest effect is on sexual desire, as expressed by sexual thoughts and fantasies. Interestingly, studies also report a general improvement in mood. This suggests that testosterone is not only a natural aphrodisiac but an antidepressant as well."

Aubrey Hill, M.D., author of *The Testosterone Solution,* asks if testosterone is a "fountain of youth." For many men, the answer is an emphatic "yes!" Testosterone replacement treatment can restore a man's testosterone level, and with it his sexuality and sense of masculinity, to that of a much younger man.

"Sexual dysfunction as well as virtually all the other symptoms of male menopause can be traced, at least in part, to an age-related decline in testosterone," say Jonathan V. Wright, M.D., and Lane

Lenard, Ph.D., authors of *Maximize Your Vitality & Potency*. "One of the brightest lights in the treatment of male menopause today is the use of testosterone replacement therapy."

Eugene R. Shippen, M.D., author of *The Testosterone Syndrome*, agrees, "Testosterone therapy has every prospect of becoming for men what estrogen therapy is now for millions of women."

That testosterone replacement therapy is a useful tool to surviving male menopause seemed to be the consensus of the researchers and scientists who met recently at the World Congress on the Aging Male in Geneva, Switzerland. Participants from more than fifty countries shared their findings on the hormonal, physical, psychological, social, and sexual aspects of men in the second half of life. More than three-quarters of the more than seven hundred participants felt that testosterone replacement was helpful to aging men and that if prescribed properly the benefits outweighed the drawbacks.

Dr. Malcolm Carruthers has treated more than two thousand men going through male menopause with testosterone and has found no adverse effects. Answering concerns that some people have about the relation between testosterone therapy and prostate cancer, Carruthers says, "Fifty years' treatment of hypogonadal patients with testosterone implants and thirty years of treatment with injections of testosterone enanthate do not show any rising incidence of prostate cancer or even benign hypertrophy."

Just as there continues to be controversy about the risks versus the benefits of estrogen and progesterone replacement for women, so too will there be concern about testosterone replacement for men.

We think of testosterone when we think of male sex hormones. But testosterone isn't the only hormone that is of importance to men. Estrogen in the male bloodstream may account for his desire, not just for sex, but for love and intimacy. Estrogen promotes receptivity and touching, qualities that both men and women value.

Lower levels of estrogen in men may relate to other life and death issues besides sex, love, and intimacy. "Men have a higher risk of heart disease, and this is presumably related to a lack of estrogen," says JoAnn E. Manson of Harvard Medical School. Many companies now are designing synthetic forms of estrogen that may help men as well as women.

Though men need some estrogen, too much can be harmful. Estrogen is produced in the male body directly from testosterone by the enzyme aromatase. A healthy young man in his twenties may have fifty times as much testosterone as estrogen while there are older men where testosterone has dropped so low and estrogen risen so high that the ratio has declined as low as three to one. These men show all the signs of low testosterone including fatigue, loss of sexual desire, depression, irritability, and anger.

High estrogen is a double-edged sword. It is not only harmful in itself, but it actually causes a further decrease in testosterone.

Causes of increased production of estrogen are:
• increased activity of the aromotase enzyme with age
• increased body fat
• lower levels of zinc and vitamin C
• cigarette smoking
• excessive alcohol intake
• use of drugs, including marijuana, amphetamines, and cocaine
• use of many common medications including aspirin, Tylenol, antidepressants, antibiotics, cholesterol lowering medications, and heart medications
• exposure to pesticides or chemicals containing xeno-estrogens (synthetic compounds that act like estrogen in the body)

So, if the man of the house is feeling less than manly these days, he may want to look over the above list and make appropriate changes.

Keeping a proper balance between testosterone and estrogen is vital as men age. There also is increasing interest in other hormones as well. William Regelson, M.D., author of *The Super-Hormone Promise,* believes that the aging process is not a normal life event but a disease in and of itself which he feels can be combated by replacing key hormones as they decline. He includes such hormones as DHEA, pregnenolone, testosterone, estrogen, thyroid hormone, human growth hormone, and melatonin.

All hormones are powerful substances. Before considering their use, a man (or a woman) should learn everything possible about the benefits and drawbacks of hormone replacement therapy, work with a health care professional trained in this area of medicine, and be willing to continue monitoring progress.

Nate is a fifty-six-year-old man, recently married for the third time. He is overweight, out of shape, drinks too much, and is depressed. He retired from a high-stress job and feels at loose ends. He has no idea what he wants to do with the rest of his life. He came to our clinic because he thought testosterone replacement therapy might be the answer to his problems. "I think it would help. I've read good things about what it can do," he said with enthusiasm, "and I'd like to give it a try."

I told him we weren't a testosterone clinic, but a health clinic, and would need to learn about the whole man so that we could work with him to come up with the right treatment for him. We had a total and free testosterone test done which showed that his levels of total testosterone where within normal limits, but his bioavailable testosterone levels were slightly low.

I told him I'd like to learn more about his eating patterns, what he was doing for exercise, and his drinking habits since they all had an effect on his overall health as well as what might be causing his symptoms. He seemed disappointed. "I know you'll probably want me to change my lifestyle, but couldn't I get started on the testosterone?"

Nate is like a lot of men who will deny that anything is changing in their lives or that they are having any problems. When they finally do wake up, they want the quick fix with the least need for any real change. Fortunately for Nate, he was willing to explore other areas than just his hormones.

Doorway #2: Let's Get Physical: Eating Well and Exercise Are Not for Sissies

Though there is value in the latest breakthroughs in hormone therapies and biological medicine, there is nothing more basic and important to men than exercise and eating. As a kid, I remember eating my spinach so that I could be healthy and strong like Popeye. Later, I ate Wheaties, the breakfast of champions. There was clearly a relationship between what we ate and the benefits of sports and exercise.

Many of us had bad eating and exercise habits early on, others have lost our good practices as we've gotten older. A few have kept healthy habits throughout our lives. Whatever our experiences, it is never too late to have a healthy life. However, many have come to believe that eating and exercise have to be painful and unpleasant. In fact, the opposite is true.

This is a time of life to eat the foods that give you gustatory delight and exercise in a way that makes you feel so good you can't wait to do it again. The time for suffering while making yourself "do the right thing" is past. Now is the time for pure pleasure. Can you handle it?

As much as we would like to deny it, there is much truth to the old adage that "we are what we eat." But with so much hype about this miracle diet or that one, it is difficult to know what path to follow. It might make sense to begin by asking the question, "what was the human body designed to eat?" Since the basic elements of our body design have not changed in the three millions years our ancestors have lived on the planet, we can look to see what diet humans ate before we began eating the Modern American Diet (which John Robbins, author of *Diet for a New America*, correctly calls MAD).

Three modern-day scientists have tackled the problem. S. Boyd Eaton, M.D. is a radiologist. Marjorie Shostak is an anthropologist and Melvin Konner, M.D., Ph.D. is one of the leading experts in the emerging field of evolutionary psychology. Together, they have written *The Paleolithic Prescription: A Program of Diet and Exercise and a Design for Living* that can tell us about the fuel the human body was designed to run on.

Though we think of our indigenous ancestors as hunter-gatherers, they would more accurately be described as gatherer-hunters. According to Eaton, Shostak, and Konner, most of our ancient diet, as much as 80 percent, was plant food—fruits and vegetables (except in the extreme north where plant foods were not available and meat was a much larger part of the diet). Meat was a delicacy that added zest (and protein) to the diet.

Other modern scientists have validated the value of this ancient diet, basically vegetarian with some meat added. The traditional Asian diet with its foundation of rice or other grains, an abundance of vegetables, fruits, beans, and legumes, limited amounts of meat and other animal foods, and virtually no dairy products is pretty close to what our ancestors ate.

Research shows that the traditional Asian diet is far healthier than ours. Proof? People in Asian countries experience lower rates of heart disease, cancer, and diabetes than do people in the U.S. In Japan, the result is the highest life expectancy in the world. The U.S. is twenty-sixth in longevity. Not wild about Asian cooking? How about Italian? The traditional Mediterranean diet with its focus on fresh vegetables and pasta is also very healthy.

Most people, particularly men, are afraid that being healthy means giving up all meat (as well as all the other foods they enjoy). However, it doesn't mean giving up things we like as much as adding more things that we like. I used to eat meat three times a day. I couldn't imagine living on less. It took me awhile to change my food preferences, but now that I have, there is so much to enjoy without having to give up anything. In the past, I loved having a good piece of prime rib at dinner (or even lunch, and leftovers for breakfast, why not?). After being off meat for awhile, I discovered I loved hot and spicy eggplant. It's better for me and I don't feel I'm missing anything, though occasionally I still enjoy fish, chicken, or beef.

Colon cancer is now the second-leading cause of cancer deaths, yet 90 percent of colon cancers are curable if caught early and 75 percent of cases are caused by dietary and lifestyle factors that are largely under our control. Eating a diet with lots of fruits and vegetables and cutting down on meat, alcohol, and tobacco products helps men's general health and also can go a long way in preventing colon cancer.

Eating well also can keep our prostate glands healthy. We now know that the prostate gland is the most frequently diseased organ of the human body.

Health and wellness expert Dr. Andrew Weil recommends a number of simple things we can do to prevent prostate problems from ever occurring, including the following:

• Drink lots of water (your urine should be light in color).

• Eat plenty of soy foods. The phytoestrogens found in soy may block the negative effects of testosterone on the prostate.

• Reduce the amount of saturated fat in your diet. According to a study done at Stanford Medical School, men who eat more than 30 grams a day of saturated fat (mostly from meat and dairy) have twice the risk of prostate cancer as do men who eat only 11 grams of saturated fat a day.

• Eat meals rich in tomatoes. A recent study conducted by the Harvard School of Public Health shows a 20 percent reduction in prostate cancer risk in men who eat tomatoes or tomato sauce four times a week and a 50 percent reduction in those who eat ten servings a week.

Along with eating well, exercise is one of the best things we can do to live long and healthy. Exercise has been a part of our lives since the beginning. "Our genetic constitution has been selected to operate within a milieu of vigorous, daily, and lifelong physical exertion," say Eaton, Shostak, and Konner. "The exercise boom is not just a fad; it is a return to 'natural' activity—the kind for which our bodies are engineered and which facilitates the proper function of our biochemistry and physiology."

Physical fitness has three main components: cardiorespiratory (aerobic) endurance, muscular strength, and flexibility.

Good cardiorespiratory endurance means that activities requiring stamina (such as soccer, swimming, running, racquetball, and basketball) can be maintained for relatively prolonged periods.

Muscular strength usually peaks between the ages of twenty and thirty, and declines steadily thereafter. Yet regular exercise can reduce the rate of decline. Strong muscles guard against injuries and exercise helps keep our bones strong and protects us against osteoporosis.

Yet, the most important aspect of our exercise program should be flexibility. Flexible bodies are limber, supple, graceful, and we might add, sexy at any age. One of the prime problems men have as we age is with our backs. This seems to be one of the side effects of having only recently, in evolutionary time, begun to walk upright.

Anyone who has ever had a back go out, and that's most all of us over age fifty, knows it is difficult to feel strong and manly, not to mention sexy, when it hurts to move. "There's definitely a strong connection between good back flexibility and great sex," says James White, Ph.D., professor emeritus at the University of California, San Diego. "A lover with a stiff back is an oxymoron."

Want some more reasons to exercise? Men's health expert Ken Goldberg, M.D., provides these reasons, aside from the obvious fact that fit people may have half as many heart attacks and strokes.

• Physical activity reduces your risk of colon cancer. According to a recent study in the journal *Cancer*, active men have much lower risk, even if they're overweight.

• Exercise protects against, and may even reverse, diabetes. In a study of twenty-two thousand doctors, those with patients who exercised regularly had 42 percent fewer cases of diabetes.

• Working out protects you from job burnout. Researchers at Tel Aviv University have found that active men are about half as likely to buckle under job stress.

• Strength training may delay aging. When a group of ninety-year-old men were put on a program of weight lifting, they increased strength by an average of 174 percent.

• Fitness helps prevent illness. A study of 8,301 employees found that unfit people were 2.5 times as likely to call in sick.

• Men who exercise are less likely to get prostate cancer. Among 20,785 Harvard alumni, only one man who burned up more than four thousand calories a week exercising got prostate cancer. Those who burned fewer than one thousand had thirty-eight cases.

• Exercise builds strong bones. Among 101 men sixty and older who took up exercise, bone density increased 19 percent on average.

• Exercisers are depression-resistant. *The American Journal of Epidemiology* reports that people who don't exercise are at "significantly greater risk of depression."

• Exercise helps you go to sleep. Duke University scientists report that men who exercise fall asleep in half the time that it takes men who don't.

• Fit people have better sex lives. When seventy-eight inactive men took up exercising three or four days a week, their frequency of intercourse increased significantly. The American Heart Association—which for the first time in twenty years has just added a heart disease risk factor to its list: inactivity—says that walking, gardening, dancing, croquet, and shuffle board are all activities that offer significant health benefits.

Doorway #3: The Psychology of Male Menopause: Healing Emotional Wounds and Deepening Our Emotional Roots

Some of the most illusive aspects of male menopause and some of the most difficult to deal with concern the psychological aspects of men's health. Though men may resist changing their diet or getting more exercise, they at least know about these things. Men are often much more cut off from their emotions and so have a more difficult time healing in these areas. It often takes some kind of a crisis to help men recognize that their emotional life is playing a key role in how well they are handling this change of life period.

Here are two stories, one from a man, the other from a woman that speak to the psychological aspects of male menopause.

I Thought Male Menopause Was a Joke

I found your book by chance in the public library. I had been joking to my friends that I was going through male menopause and didn't even know it exists.

I have only just begun to read your book and everything you say is right on target. I was beginning to think I was losing it. I had lost my zest for life. I kept losing my temper. Little things that seemed of no consequence would set me off. I found myself yelling at my wife, which is not at all like me. My wife says she thinks I may be depressed. After reading the section on the differences between male depression and female depression, I think she may be right.

I told my wife what I was reading and how accurate it was. She thought it was great. She had even told me a year ago to go see a counselor after I had told her about my insecurities. I didn't listen to her then. I thought I could handle it all myself.

To tell you the truth, I've never been the kind of guy who thought much about my emotions. I've always been a pretty happy-go-lucky person. If there is something wrong I just handle it on my own. But this is something I can't seem to get through. The more I try to get to the bottom of it, the more confused I get. I alternate between wanting to run away from my life and start over somewhere and just wanting to ignore things and go on like business as usual.

I also have been having more thoughts about my past. I think about my father and the things he never gave me. He was never around and when he was, he treated me like I was one of his possessions. I don't think he really respected me as a person. I still carry a lot of anger.

After reading your book, I feel it's time to deal with these issues. I thought time heals all wounds. But I see that some things need to be taken care of or they just get covered over and fester over the years.

Thanks for giving me some guidance and the knowledge that I'm not the only guy going through this.

I'll let you know how it turns out.

Stephen

Points of understanding:

• Sometimes, the best approach to helping a man deal with the emotional aspects of male menopause is to take an indirect route: he finds the book in a library; someone sends him a copy for Christmas; his friends mention it and he finds an article on the subject.

• Often, we don't see the problems in ourselves but when we read it or hear about it in others, it's like a mirror held up where we can see it.

• A woman often will notice the emotional changes and point them out to the man. At first, he may deny there is anything there, that she is imagining things, that things are fine. Later, he may acknowledge there are emotional problems, but may feel he can handle them himself. Finally, he often recognizes that he needs to reach out for help and that help is available.

• It takes patience and perseverance to keep at it, even when he seems most resistant. Sometimes the best approach is to sit back and do nothing, waiting for him to discover what he needs to find.

• Quite often, this time of life pulls us back to unhealed emotional elements from the past. It is one of the reasons men resist male menopause. No one likes to feel pain and many have spent years trying to forget about painful experiences. However, pain signals old wounds that never healed and continue to cause problems in the present. Returning to the past can allow us to heal completely and put the past to rest so we can go on with the future.

My Husband Is an Alcoholic and Going through Male Menopause

My husband is now fifty-two years old and was an alcoholic for many years before he began going to AA meetings in 1994. I really started to believe our marriage was finally going to take a turn for the better. Our four children started to get closer to him and the fights that had caused so much strain began to diminish. But in January, he walked out on us. He is now living with a younger woman who also belongs to AA.

I should have seen it coming. We had been having sexual problems for some time. He also told me he has had nightmares about his drinking days and even told me he thought he was going through "the change." I just laughed. He also had mood swings and seemed tired all the time. I believe he may have been having memory problems. He would say something to me and when I'd ask him about it later, he would say he never said it.

Now I'm taking his concerns seriously, I hope it isn't too late.
Mary Beth

Points of understanding:

• For many men, alcohol or other drugs have been used to keep uncomfortable emotions out of consciousness. When this goes on for years, it can lead to dependency and addiction.

• When a man stops drinking, there is hope that life will begin to get better for him and his family. Generally, this is true, but it also releases emotions that have long been buried and need to be dealt with.

• When this occurs during the male menopause years, there is a need for particular sensitivity and awareness. Men need support, but are often faced with indifference, anger, or ridicule.

• Men who have inflicted pain on others need to recognize that healing will take time. Women who have felt damaged by the emotional abuse need to understand that he and you may need continuing support through this change of life period.

Depression: The Silent Killer of Men

Depression is one of the most common symptoms of male menopause and is closely related to the lowering of sexual desire and function that also are hallmarks of male menopause. A man whose sex life is on the rocks is likely to be depressed; and a man who is depressed is likely to have serious problems with his sex life. Yet, most men who suffer from depression aren't even aware that they have it. They often don't recognize themselves when they hear the classic symptoms of major depression such as persistent sad moods, recurrent thoughts of death, diminished ability to think or concentrate, feeling worthless, sleeping too much, low energy, loss of pleasure in life's activities, and/or significant weight loss or gain.

Women often express their depression by focusing inward and blaming themselves. Men often express their depression by focusing outward and blaming others. This was true in my own life. It wasn't until I recognized that my irritability, anger, and blame were manifestations of depression that I was finally able to ask for help and receive treatment. I know the recognition that I was suffering from depression saved my marriage and very likely saved my life.

There are now more effective treatments for depression and the emotional aspects of male menopause. Men should have no more reluctance to being treated for depression than they would being treated for high blood pressure. There are medications, herbs, exercises, stress reduction techniques, and counseling available. Don't wait until the problems get serious to seek help. Overcoming depression may be the greatest gift a man can get in his lifetime.

In many ways, the male menopause passage is a "dark night of the soul." It is a time to go down and feel our emotions, to feel the pain from the past, and to deal with unfinished business so it can be healed. It also can be a time of rebirth, a time of letting go of old dramas and traumas so we can feel the love that awaits us in the second half of life.

Doorway #4: The Interpersonal Level: New Opportunities for Intimacy and Love

Dr. Paul Pearsall has been studying the relationship between the body, mind, and spirit for many years. He is the author of many books on sex, love, and intimacy including the *New York Times* bestseller *Super Marital Sex*. Unlike many experts in the field, Dr. Pearsall is not afraid to share his personal experiences going through male menopause.

In his recent book, *The Heart's Choice*, he says, "Ten years ago in late fall, I remember thinking how the crinkled dry leaves seemed to reflect my own vague sense of internal decay. I felt weak, had an almost constant headache, and sweated so heavily at night that the bed was soaked in the morning. I often told my wife that there was some form of toxic energy in me that I could not describe, but when I told my doctors about this sense of impending doom that I seemed to be experiencing in my heart, they responded that their tests showed nothing they considered abnormal and that I was just under stress from my clinical work. My brain accepted the diagnosis, but my heart remained very worried."

It turned out Dr. Pearsall's heart was right. The doctors finally found that he was suffering from an advanced form of cancer. If the cancer had been caught sooner, he would have been saved years of suffering. He was not saved by science, but by his most intimate relationship.

I am still moved by Pearsall's description that I reported in my book, *Male Menopause*. "I had never known such helplessness and terror," Pearsall remembers. "I was blind and unable to move. Even my eyelids would not open in response to my efforts to cling to my tenuous connection with the world. I had just been taken to intensive care following surgery for cancer that had spread through my body and into my bones. I struggled to breathe and to move any part of my body, and I felt totally isolated and alone.

"I heard the words of a doctor pronouncing, 'I think we've lost him.' At my time of helplessness and isolation, my wife, Celest, brought me back from death's door and reconnected me with life. I felt the warmth of her breath against my cheek, the wetness of her tears falling gently on my eyelids, and the soothing and reassuring comfort of her fingers tracing along my arms, chest, and the scars that lined my abdomen. 'I love you. I'm here. You'll make it, sweetheart. We'll make it together like we always do,' she cried softly in my ear."

His wife's love gave him something that modern medicine, with all its technological wizardry, could not. It gave him a reason to live. "Like the electric paddles that shock a heart back to normal rhythm and bring a patient back to life, my wife's words seemed to be the catalyst for a flood of memories we had made together," said Pearsall. "As I lay near death, it was not my life that passed before my eyes—it was our life."

I had a similar experience not too long ago when I was in the hospital having a rare tumor removed. Not only did I have my wife, Carlin, at my bedside before and after the surgery, but I had one of my best friends, Tom, who gave me the kind of male support I needed. If we have family with us during this time of life, we are blessed. If we have close friends, we are doubly blessed.

In the first half of our lives, our friendships and love lives are often passionate, but don't have the depth that many years together brings. In the first half, love and intimacy are not touched with possibility of death. In the second half, death is a companion that we must all get to know. I would never have chosen to have a life-threatening tumor, but having been close to death, I know he is a friend, not someone to be feared. He allows us to live life to the fullest and remember that we never know when he may come for us. He teaches us that we must live and love today as if it were our last.

This is a time for healing our relationships and deepening our connections. The media may portray men as being obsessed with sex from birth to death, but real men know that love and intimacy with a partner, care and support from our families, and the connection with close friends are what makes this stage of life worth living. This requires some of the most difficult work a man and woman can experience in their lives. Often, good counseling can be of help. If there's a spark of life in your relationship, never give up on it. Seeing it glow and burst into flame is worth all the hard work.

Doorway #5: Sex on the Second Mountain: It Gets Better If We Let It

As Bruce Handy said in his cover story for *Time* magazine, "The Viagra Craze," "What else can one say but *Vrooom!* Cheap gas, strong economy, erection pills—what a country! What a time to be alive!" The time was 1998, specifically March 28, 1998, the day Viagra was approved by the FDA to help men with their flagging erections.

Up until that time, erectile dysfunction, or impotence as it was known, was the secret men kept from their doctors, their partners, even from themselves. Now all of a sudden, erectile dysfunction had come out of the closet and everyone was talking about the little blue pill that instantly brought erections back into a man's life.

We are a quick-fix society. We all want the magic pill that will make everything right in our world. Viagra's popularity taps that belief that we can improve our sexual lives quickly and easily. In the thirty-five years I have been working with men and women, there have been many "magic sexual potions" trumpeted in the media. There seem to be an equal number of "magic new diets" that are sure to melt the fat right off our bodies without pain or strain. I've learned that there is no free lunch, no instant cures for a lifetime of poor eating practices, and no way to regain a healthy sex life overnight.

Viagra, and other drugs that will be touted as the new "passion pill," is not magic. Though there are indications that it is safe and effective, we don't yet have long-term results. We have only to remember thalidomide, which was first deemed safe and later shown to cause serious birth defects, or more recently fen-phen, which was thought to be a miracle drug for losing weight and was later withdrawn because of fears that it caused heart problems. I recommend caution to those who would jump on the technology bandwagon, for Viagra or for any of the upcoming bio-tech breakthroughs.

Viagra won't repair a relationship torn apart by shame, fear, anger, and doubt. It takes time and often professional counseling to rebuild a damaged relationship. It may restore erections if passion is present. But desire comes from love and connection which are at the foundation of our sexual lives. This came clear to me once again as I read a recent survey.

It was billed as the most important and accurate sex survey in more than forty years, "surpassing all previous sexuality surveys—including Kinsey, Masters and Johnson, and the Hite Report." The findings were published in two volumes, one for the general public, (*Sex in America: A Definitive Study*) and the other for social scientists, counselors, and health professionals (*The Social Organization of Sexuality*).

Published in 1994, the chapter titles of the popular version give an idea of the material covered: Sex in America, The Sex Survey, Who Are Our Sex Partners, Finding a Partner, How Many Sex Partners Do We Have?, Practices and Preferences, Masturbation and Erotica, Homosexual Partners, Sexually Transmitted Diseases, AIDS, Forced Sex, and Sex and Society.

As I read through the material, I wondered, where is love and intimacy discussed? Not much in evidence, according to this "definitive" book. The index gave few listings for either "love" or "intimacy." More space was given to a discussion of "forced sex" and rape.

It seems that sex in America has become like white sugar—highly refined, very intense, found everywhere, compulsively sought after, and ultimately empty of nourishment. Sex, according to author George Leonard, who has written extensively on the subject, has become "an activity, a field of study, an entity that somehow seems to exist almost entirely separated from life."

For men, sex on the First Mountain is often focused on "how much" and "how fast." William, a sixty-four-year-old man, voiced it this way, "When I was in my twenties and thirties, I wanted as much sex as I could get and I wanted it now. I often felt deprived. No matter how much my wife was available (when we had children, she was busy a lot), I wanted more.

"After I reached forty-five or fifty things began to change. At first I thought I was losing it. I wasn't as turned on all the time as I used to be. My erections were more sensitive to how I was feeling. If I didn't feel loved or didn't feel in a loving mood, I lost my erection and that was that. I wanted to get back that 'instant turn on.'

"But the more I thought about it—and I have to admit, it was my wife that helped me see it this way—I realized that I was moving into a new kind of sexuality, one that isn't driven so much by my hormones and the desire to reproduce. When I stopped fighting the feeling it was really quite nice. We still make love and enjoy all the old feelings of passion we felt in our youth, but we also make love with just a touch of the hand, a look of recognition, a smile. I never thought I would say it, but I feel like we are making love just being together or even just thinking about each other.

"I thought I would do anything to get back the sexuality of my youth. Now I know that the sexuality I have is what I want at this time of my life. Its more expansive, more enjoyable, passionate in a more deeply loving way, more intimate, gentler, and more joyful."

Men who cling exclusively to a "youthful sexuality" will be increasingly disappointed as their First Mountain sexuality, like their youth, slips away. Men who are willing to the risk having a new kind of sexuality emerge will find that their sex lives expand and grow in ways they never imagined.

Doorway #6: Developing a Social Life for the Ages: Men Need Others More Than Ever

When my first wife and I divorced, I made a terrible discovery. I found that somewhere along the way I had lost my social connections. She had become the one who arranged social get-togethers. She sent out birthday cards and made constant phone calls, which I hated at the time, but realized were the ways relationships were kept alive. She was surrounded by women friends who offered her support to get through the difficulties surrounding our separation and divorce.

When I looked around, I saw a lot of emptiness. I realized that I felt ashamed that my marriage had failed and I was reluctant to talk to the friends I did have. I tried to pretend that everything was all right. I didn't work and I began to become dangerously withdrawn. A friend told me he was starting a men's group and asked me if I wanted to check it out. I refused at first, but seeing my ex-wife get so much support from her women's group, I was convinced that it was worth a try.

That decision changed, perhaps even saved, my life. For the first time, I felt I was able to open up and talk about my anger and pain, my guilt and shame, as well as my hopes and dreams with others who understood and could empathize because they had been there themselves. The weekly meetings became the cornerstone of a revitalized life for me.

Throughout my first marriage, my life had revolved around my family and my work. My work, though satisfying, didn't mean much if I didn't have a family to come home to. With my marriage on the rocks and my life as a single father staring me in the face, I realized how precarious my support system had been.

It wasn't until I joined the men's group that I realized how important men friends were in my life. As we got to know each other and told our stories, listened, empathized, laughed, occasionally shed a tear or two, we captured something most of us had never had. We found a deep connection with other men.

Most of us had grown up with fathers who were absent through divorce, desertion, death, or overwork. We had brothers who we competed with for attention and love in our families. We had buddies who disappeared over the years or let us down when we needed them. We had men at work who we worried were after our jobs and men in the world who we worried were after our women. We didn't trust other men and we didn't trust ourselves not to "do it to them, before they did it to us."

Learning to break down the barriers and trust other men was the most important work I could do. I believe that men who aren't able to do that, who don't learn to develop close male friendships, are much more likely to become depressed, get sick, and die too soon. We know that men die sooner and contract every major disease at rates much high than women. Our greater social isolation may well be the reason.

A survey conducted by the Third Age Wellness Center in 1999 validated the difference between male social support and what females experience.

Men receive support from the following sources:

    68 percent spouse

    10 percent relative

    10 percent friend

    2 percent co-worker

    10 percent none

Women receive support from the following sources:

    25 percent spouse

    40 percent relative

    30 percent friend

    2 percent co-worker

    3 percent none

The first thing that stands out is that men rely on their spouse for the great majority of their support. They put most of their eggs in that one basket. Women, on the other hand, get most of their support from relatives and friends. If a man is having trouble with his wife or gets divorced, he loses his support system. If a woman is having similar difficulties, her support system remains intact. Also, more than twice as many men as women have no support at all in their lives.

After being in my first men's group for five years, I moved out of the area. Recognizing the benefits of men's support, I immediately joined another group. I have been with that same group of men for more than twenty years now. I'm convinced that the support I get is the prime reason I have been able to develop a solid, healthy relationship with a woman and maintain my health and well-being as I have gotten older.

There are men's organizations and groups that are providing support for men. Many have heard of the Million Man March in Washington, D.C., and the meetings of the Promise Keepers. There are also gatherings of men under the banner of the Mankind Project (the New Warrior Weekends) and the Sterling Men's Weekends.

There is a recognition that men need the support of other men, not just for sports or for a beer after work, but for intimacy, care, and love. Too many men are dying because they haven't learned how to reach out to other men. One of the greatest gifts a man can give to himself is the gift of other men in his life. It's never too late to start.

Doorway #7: Spirit: The Central Source of Our Lives

Like love, spirit is an essential aspect of our lives that is very difficult to define. "Any journalist worth his or her salt," says former persidential advisor and journalist Bill Moyers, "knows the real story today is to define what it means to be spiritual." This is the biggest story—not only of the decade but of the century.

As we begin into the twenty-first century, spirituality seems to have emerged as a major focus in many people's lives.

• There is an increased interest in myth and ritual. Carl Jung and Joseph Campbell have been rediscovered and their writings have taught many about the place of spirituality in ancient and modern cultures.

• East has met West as religious and spiritual practices from Japan, China, India, and Tibet have spread to the U.S.

• Martial arts such as Aikido, Kung Fu, Judo, and Tai Chi are found everywhere and their spiritual basis is widely taught.

• Alcoholics Anonymous and similar twelve-step programs are recognizing that giving up spirits cannot occur without a reconnection with Spirit.

• Therapists are exploring the relationship between spirituality and psychotherapy and have recognized the importance of spiritual healing to the healing of the total person. Mind/Body/Spirit healing are seen as working together for the betterment of the client and his family.

• Medical pioneers are showing that people get sick less often and heal faster if they have a spiritual practice in their lives. Prayer is being recognized as a scientifically valid method of healing.

• Feminist spirituality has rediscovered the Goddess and has introduced feminine vocabulary in viewing the Divine.

• Men, as well as women, have reconnected with indigenous cultural traditions and have rediscovered the spiritual traditions of Native Americans and other peoples.

• The ecological movement has gone beyond a material focus on saving natural resources and also embraces a spiritual belief in the sacredness of all life.

• The old warfare between science and religion has ended and a new synthesis is beginning. New connections between such "hard" sciences as physics and the "soft" spiritual and mystical traditions are being made.

• Even Fortune 500 companies are introducing meditation, poetry, and spiritual practices into the workplace, recognizing that workers need more than money and retirement benefits to feel successful.

Why is there so much attention being paid to spirituality lately? Clearly there is a great need and what worked in the past may not be what people need now. Maybe you have lost connection with the spiritual tradition in which you were raised or never really made a connection in the first place. Maybe you were turned off by the hypocrisy you found. Maybe you hoped that science and technology would find the answers to the questions of right and wrong, meaning and truth. Maybe you've been searching for some kind of religious or spiritual tradition that can comfort you in times of turmoil.

You may have had to confront some new realities in the second half of life. Perhaps your success or failure at work has caused you to reach out for new meaning or purpose. Perhaps the ending of a long-time relationship has brought you to question the meaning of love and commitment. Perhaps you've become estranged from a grown child and you wonder what went wrong when you raised him. Perhaps your parents have gotten sick and you must decide how to take care of them. Perhaps you've been present at the death of a parent and had the terror and ecstasy of looking into the eyes of God as you said good-bye and held them in your arms. Perhaps you've dealt with illness in your own life and had to confront your own ending.

All these experiences force us to look for the ultimate meaning in our lives. As we are running the base paths of life, as my father saw it, and make the turn around second base, there are questions that draw our attention. We want to know who we are, what we've really contributed to the world, and what is the meaning of our lives. This is the realm of spirituality. But for each of us that realm is different.

As Sam Keen, author of *Hymns to an Unknown God: Awakening the Spirit in Everyday Life*, says, "Just as there is no universal diet that is healthy for all persons, just as Jack Sprat could eat no fat and his wife could eat no lean, no single spiritual diet will be nourishing for everyone. The ways we metabolize meaning are as profoundly different as the ways we metabolize food. Some thrive on a diet of elaborate symbols and will be nourished by high church liturgy, an intricate Tibetan tanka, or a Jungian mandala. Others are allergic to excessive theological ritual and will do much better with Quaker silence or Zen meditation."

The search for spirit, for God, Keen says, "Is ultimately the quest to know ourselves in our heights and depths. It is the task of every man and woman and of every heroic journey to go beyond our certitudes and doubts, beyond our sure knowledge and understanding, in the direction of an ever-unfolding truth. It was, is, and always will be the greatest human adventure."

Helping Men Deal with All Seven Doorways of Male Menopause

I think of male menopause as offering a man the opportunity to learn about this adventure that can only begin at midlife. All the changes we experience are wake-up calls to let us know it is time to embark. Each aspect is like a doorway that a man can enter. Just as there is no universal spiritual path, neither is there one path through male menopause.

When I work with a man and his family, I am alert to what doorway he is most ready to enter. For some men, it is clear that the sexual doorway beckons to them. Others are first drawn to the hormonal or physical aspects. Yet, others are concerned with the psychological or interpersonal sides or the social or spiritual realms.

Wherever a man is ready to begin, I'm ready to meet him. Ultimately, each doorway leads into a large courtyard where all aspects come together. The journey can't be hurried. Its purpose is to help us let go of the things that keep us bound to the past, help us decide what qualities and practices we need to take with us, and what we have to look forward to in the future.

Chapter 6

Super-Adulthood
The Best Is Yet to Come

Remember that male menopause, like its female counterpart, is a major life transition. Far from being the beginning of the end as many fear, it is really the end of the beginning. It closes out the first stage of our journey on earth and prepares us for the next, more interesting stage.

The Three Ages of Man: Moving into Super-Adulthood

At the Third Age Wellness Center, we divide the life cycle into three parts. The first age, childhood, extends from birth to around age twenty-one. The second age, adulthood, extends from age eighteen to fifty. The third age, super-adulthood, extends from forty-five to one hundred or more.

We call it super-adulthood for a number of reasons. As we continue to extend the life span, it has become the longest part of our lives. It is also a time when we are free to pursue our soul work, to express the depths of who we are in the world and what we are here to contribute.

A New Awakening

John, fifty-five, is just at the beginning of his super-adulthood and is learning to appreciate the opportunities that come with it.

I felt like I was awakening from a long sleep or coming though years living in the fog. When I first started to see you, I didn't know what was going on with me. I knew I was under a lot of stress on the job, and having my twelve-year-old daughter move in with us turned out to be quite an adjustment.

It's only looking back now that I can see a little more clearly what I've been through. I remember you told me about the seven aspects of male menopause. I have to be honest and say I thought it was all a bunch of bologna when I first heard about it.

When I thought about menopause, I thought about what my wife, Betsy, was beginning to go through. If I was aware of it at all, which I tried not to be, all I felt was the fear that my wife was going to get old and dried up, and our sex life would go down the tubes. That's what seemed to have happened with my parents.

When I first heard about it, I thought male menopause was a joke. The only problem I could see at the time was an unruly daughter who pushed us to the limits and beyond. I had more interest in getting her situation fixed than trying to figure out what might be happening to me. The problem was that fixing the situation with her didn't seem to work. My wife and I got more and more frustrated and I got more and more irritable and angry.

The counseling you gave us helped with many of the interpersonal problems we were experiencing. It took me a number of years to be willing to deal with my own issues. I began to see how frustrated I had become and how much I was blaming my wife, my boss, my family, and my friends. When I finally admitted that the problem was inside me, I felt overwhelmed with shame.

For a long time, I couldn't get past the feeling that I was a failure in life. I wasn't advancing in my job like I had hoped, I felt distant from my wife and family, I had lost interest in going out and being together. I just wanted to be left alone. I retreated into watching sports. When I wasn't working, I was glued to the TV. I knew Betsy missed me, but I couldn't face her.

You helped me break out of my shame and I finally could admit I had slipped into a depression. For a long time, I was unwilling to even consider medication, but I knew I needed something more than counseling could provide. You helped me see that depression was a disease like any other and was very treatable. I gave antidepressant medication a try and it seemed to be the missing piece for putting my emotional life back on an even keel.

As I felt less depressed, my interest in Betsy returned. I wanted to make up for all the lost sexual opportunities I had missed. It took me awhile to understand that Betsy had withdrawn and she needed time to regain her feelings for me. I didn't realize how much my anger had hurt her and how wounded she felt. It took us some time to rekindle our connection. At first we felt like teenagers, awkward and tense. The old feeling of ease had deserted us. Now we had to learn to be intimate all over again.

I found I was having difficulty getting and maintaining an erection, which added to the tension. You helped me understand that there were causes and once we found them, we could fix the problem. At the time, I was too overwhelmed with fear and shame. That's when I dropped out of counseling and slipped back into depression. Betsy's support got us through that time. She was so kind and loving. She kept telling me that we would get through this together. She didn't make demands on me, just held me when I was down on myself.

I stopped taking the medications, but that didn't help with the erections like I hoped it would. Finally, I came back for counseling and you helped me find a different medication that helped. We tried Viagra which did me some good. But it was the testosterone that seemed to restore the vitality and excitement that had been missing. The doctor at the clinic found that I was pretty low, and prescribed the patch which gave me renewed vigor in my life.

I realized, though, that no medication can help heal a relationship. The real healing for our sex lives came from the support I received from Betsy and my letting go of so much of my self-shame and blame that kept me from accepting her love.

There was so much that helped. The exercise program you prescribed and the change in diet made a big difference. The men's group I joined gave me a place to open up and be myself. I hadn't had so much fun since I was ten years old and had a group of buddies that hung out together. I hadn't realized how much I missed that until the men's group helped me see how important other guys are in our lives.

My involvement in the men's group led to greater involvement in the community. A number of us began working at the local high school to help boys at risk before there were problems. I found I had a real knack for that sort of thing. I really liked meeting with these young men, listening to their hopes and dreams, and sharing some of my life experience. Rather than sitting at home watching sports on TV, I've started playing ball with the boys and coaching them. I've even entertained the idea of going back to school and getting a degree in counseling or educational psychology. I used to think it was too late to start a new career. Now I know it's never too late.

Betsy and I have been going to a number of different spiritual events in the community. Neither one of us feel connected to traditional religion, but we both are feeling a hunger for something beyond the realm of human understanding. We haven't found all the answers we are seeking, but the questions keep us humble. There was a community sing the other night, where all different churches and groups in the town came together. It was wonderful. It didn't matter what religion you were. There was a place where we could celebrate being human.

It feels so wonderful to be alive now. For me, male menopause makes a great deal of sense. I've been through it, and now look forward to the next stage of the journey. When I began going through male menopause, it felt like everything was falling apart in me. Now I realize I was being stripped of all the old parts that were no longer needed. I feel like a space craft that has shed the booster rockets that launched it, and without carrying the dead weight can fly farther out into space. Whatever the next phase of life has to offer, I'm going for it!

Dealing With Death: an Opportunity for Life

Carlin had gone to Portland to join two of her oldest friends at their fortieth high school reunion. When she left, I jokingly told her not to have a fling with any of her high school sweethearts. I trusted her completely, but I'll probably never be so secure that I don't have a little bit of insecurity when my wife is having fun with friends and I'm not around.

Since it was a quick trip, fly up, class bash, and fly back, I hadn't expected to hear from her. But when I heard her voice on the phone I knew something was wrong. She had said she was going to stop to see her Mom who was recovering from a bout of food poisoning and I had a quick flash that maybe her Mom had gotten worse. I wasn't prepared for what I heard.

"Mom has cancer," Carlin said, her voice sad, but strong. "We're doing some more tests tomorrow, but it looks like it's spread and the doctors don't think it's curable."

I was stunned and scared about what I would hear next. "I want to bring her back with me and have her stay with us." I swallowed hard. "What do you think?"

There wasn't time for me to think. All I knew was that there was an emergency and my wife needed me, and somewhere at the back of my mind, I sensed her mother needed me, too.

"Of course," I said. "Bring her as soon as you're ready. I'll start getting the house fixed up."

"I love you," she said.

"I love you, too. Tell Bess I'll be thinking about her."

When I was younger, I dreaded the thought of taking care of an older person. I was glad my mother had insisted that she never wanted to be a burden and when it was her time to go, she died very quickly.

As the reality began to sink in, I remembered Carlin's words, "What do you think?" I realized I was thinking a lot. What if her mother is in pain? How will I deal with that? What if she is bedridden and I have to feed her, bathe her, deal with her toilet needs? What if she goes on and on, losing more of her humanity day by day, while her body is kept alive? I've faced death, but what will it be like if I have to deal with prolonged illness in my own life? I'm not sure I'm ready for that.

I realized I was thinking myself into a frenzy. A wise friend gave me some sound advice. "Don't worry about what you are going to do in the future. Wait until she gets here and just bring who you are to each situation that arises. You've got a lot to give to Bess and she has a lot to give to you." I felt calmer immediately. I realized that one of the great gifts of the menopause passage was dealing with death.

Once she arrived and got settled, life took on its own routine. Carlin did most of the day-to-day care. I knew if I was going to give what I could I had to be totally present. I couldn't hold back out of fear. I had a heart-to-heart talk with Bess and told her that I was truly glad she was with us and I needed her to be totally honest with me. If there was something she wanted, she should ask me. If I was doing something she didn't want, to tell me.

In the last days of her life, I received the greatest gift anyone can receive. I spent many hours simply sitting with her and holding her hand. We looked into each other's eyes and it was like looking into the eyes of God. I saw complete and unconditional love and peace. There was no fear or anger. I had been given a glimpse through the veil to the other side and knew I need never fear death. It was only the next stage.

Since then, I've told everyone I know not to shy away from someone who is getting close to death. Be with them. It will be the greatest gift you can ever receive. It's the only thing that can help combat the fear so many of us have about aging.

In a society like ours that values people for what they do more than for who they are, those who can no longer produce in the market economy are viewed as useless. "I have learned that a culture which equates material possessions with success," says Sharon Curtin, author of *Nobody Ever Died of Old Age*, "and views the frantic, compulsive consumer as the perfect citizen, can afford little space for the aged human being. They are past competing, they are out of the game. We live in a culture which endorses what has been called 'human obsolescence.' After adolescence, obsolescence. To the junk heap, the nursing home, the retirement village, the 'Last Resort.'"

Being with Bess during her last days showed me that death is not something to be feared, but accepted and honored. Male menopause is the preparation period for living life fully in the second half. It's only when we give up on our lives, when we feel we have nothing to offer, that the thought of death shakes us with fear.

The Fountain of Youth or the Joy of Eldering: Which Would You Choose?

More than anything else, Robert wanted the red sports car he had been eyeing for more than a year. "I deserve it," he told me during one of our recent therapy sessions. "I've been working hard on my business. We just closed the biggest deal of my career and I want a reward."

Robert has the boyish good looks of the perpetual adolescent, though he just turned forty. He and his girlfriend, Judith, have been together for two years, but Robert has been unable to commit. "Women are so unpredictable," he told me, "and I'm not sure she's the one. As soon as I think it might be great to settle down and get married, she starts to get closer and I begin to feel smothered."

Robert had been concerned about his graying hair, the difficulty he was having keeping his weight under control, and a general feeling of lethargy. He had heard about a health clinic in Palm Springs, California, and had brought in their literature before deciding to go.

The first sheet out of the packet was a reprint from the magazine *Hippocrates* with an article about the new field of antiaging medicine. The headline for the article said much about what is being sold to older men: "The latest antiaging drug is cheap, convenient, and makes you feel like a kid again."

There are many things we can do to make the second half of our lives joyful and productive. I don't believe that one of them is to return to our youth. In fact, as long as we seek youth as the goal of second adulthood, we sacrifice the joy of being real men. There is something much finer that lies ahead for us than perpetual youth.

Those who focus on staying young easily become addicted to the next product that seems to offer an image of youth. Robert didn't buy the sports car. In counseling, he began to realize that the hunger he was feeling would not really be satisfied with another new toy. He realized that trying to fulfill all the desires of youth was a never ending quest and could not lead to contentment.

Though we often have a difficult time accepting it, the nutrients of life that we need for the second half are different than those that nourished us in the first. That's why those who cling to youth in the second half of life often become hooked on trying to stay forever young. Rather than find what is truly satisfying, many keep trying to fill the void with more of the same. For these men, too much is never enough.

Seeing men in the second half of their lives desperately holding on to the glories of youth is like watching animals in the zoo. There is a compulsive restlessness about their behavior. They go back and forth from one side of their cage to the other, anxious and at the same time bored.

There is a parable in the Talmud in which a traveler comes upon an old man planting a carob tree. "When will the tree bear fruit?" asks the traveler. "Oh, perhaps in seventy years," replies the old man. "Do you expect to live to eat the fruit of that tree?" "No," says the old man, "but I didn't find the world desolate when I entered it, and as my father planted for me before I was born, so do I plant for those who come after me."

Many of us have come to feel that we have nothing worth giving, no nourishment that anyone really needs. If you believe this, you are mistaken. I tell you truthfully, you are needed. There is no one else on this earth that can give what you can give. We are each put on the planet to offer our special gifts and what we have to offer is unique and precious. "What we do is nothing but a drop in the ocean," Mother Teresa reminds us, "but if we didn't do it, the ocean would be one drop less."

Albert Schweitzer, who spent fifty years of his life serving his fellow man in the oppressive heat of the African jungle, providing medical aid to those most desperately in need, said something which can guide us all at this time of our lives, "I don't know what your destiny will be, but one thing I do know; the only ones among you who will be really happy are those who have sought and found how to serve."

Many of us hold ourselves back because we feel inadequate to the task. We feel that we have done nothing in life to influence others in a positive way. We compare ourselves to others and find that we fall short. "If I had the compassion of a Schweitzer I'd have something to give," we tell ourselves. "If I had the strength of Mother Teresa, I'd have something worthy to offer others."

The truth is, we have the only gift we will ever need, the gift of ourselves. All of our heroes have flaws. So do we. But we can all give of ourselves to those who need the special gift that only we can offer.

He and She: Looking Back on the Menopause Passage

Jack, age sixty-nine, is a retired school superintendent. His wife Margaret, age sixty-eight, is a retired nurse. They have three grown children and two grandchildren. Although like all couples they have had their ups and downs, their thirty-nine-year marriage has been happy and successful. Looking back on the years between forty and fifty-five, Margaret had this to say:

Margaret's Story

Things improved greatly during those years. Jack was depressed throughout his thirties, mourning the loss of his childhood dreams of success and feeling tied down by the family. In his forties, we both began to feel some sense of power in the community and that expanded into a sense of command over our family, jobs, and outside activities. Our children were all in school, which allowed me to work outside the home. The added income gave us both a greater sense of freedom.

During this time, Jack ran for the school board and won twice. This position sustained him during a six-month period between jobs. When he finally got a job again as a school superintendent, it allowed him more discretion over how he spent his workday.

For me it was a time where my creative energy burst forth. It was like a second adolescence with wide shifts of mood, but free of the pains from all the mistakes and ignorance of youth.

Menopause, for me, was a rather smooth transition. I think male menopause was much more difficult for Jack. Women are used to dealing with it and getting support from others. Men tend to have more denial and are more fixated on keeping their image of strength and control. If they have been successful in work and spent many years in the public eye, like Jack, it is even more difficult to adjust to the change.

Probably the most difficult change in our whole lives together was when Jack retired. It was a bigger disruption than the birth of our first child. He had been working since he was a teenager and all of a sudden he had no role, no title, no job definition. He became very dependent on me, almost like a child. He couldn't think clearly. He lost his initiative, and needed me to show him how things worked around the house. It just wasn't like him.

Though we had both worked through most of our married life, the house was always my domain. When Jack came home, he tried to take over. It's understandable really. He was used to being in charge, particularly when he was around women. He'd spent forty years being surrounded by secretaries, research assistants, and waitresses, all female, all focused on being supportive of his needs.

I was totally unprepared for this. The stress became so great I literally became ill and was in bed for three months. When I felt enough energy to get out of bed, I took a trip to visit friends. One told me I ought to leave Jack. If I believed it would go on like it had, I might have been tempted. But I knew Jack needed to find his own structure and he finally did.

He joined a men's group where there were a number of younger men. For the first time in his life he began to hear stories of men's pain. One day he came home crying. I'd never seen him cry before. I asked him about it and his response touched my heart. He told me he was thinking about himself when he was nine years old. I could tell he was in pain, remembering what he didn't receive from his father. It was a real breakthrough for him and for us, too.

Jack's Story

The first ten years of our marriage, from the time I was thirty until I was forty, were accompanied by some depression. When forty came around, I had already come to terms with much of this, so the social fears about turning forty had less impact than with other men I knew. Having children and watching my family grow gave me a sense of accomplishment.

I also had good friends and satisfying job prospects. Perhaps marrying late had something to do with my greater comfort of life at this time. However, although my depression lifted, there was still a great deal of emotional pain as I got older. I have always had an active fantasy life and I do recall sadness at giving up early dreams that I now realize were totally unrealistic. From the time I was six years old I wanted to be a U.S. senator. However, I think those dreams gave me some goals that did serve to motivate me. I found ways of serving in other capacities.

But sometimes I didn't feel I had really found my true profession. I had taken some jobs more out of necessity than real desire. I felt a sadness when I had to acknowledge to myself that I could not go back and start over to remake my dreams in some other form that would be more workable. As the Dutch proverb goes: "...too late, too smart..."

I think, if I had it to do over, I would have started earlier in life with an interest that I could master that would carry me through in later years. I would have been less concerned about what others thought of me and more concerned about following my own interests and desires.

There were times I thought I had lost my chance to do something really great in the world. Recently, I realized that we can have great impact in small ways.

When I joined the men's group, my life was transformed. For the first time in my life, I really felt I had something to offer younger men. I could listen to them without judgment. I could hug them with genuine warmth. Young men would call me and we'd spend hours on the phone, mostly just sharing feelings. We would often meet for breakfast at a local cafe. I think I found my calling. I've become a mentor.

I see myself much more now in relation to my community, more as a giver than a receiver. I found that finding a place to pass on my life experiences to younger men is one of the prime rewards of life. At the same time, it is important to recognize the spiritual roots of my life, so I can really connect with all life in a non-threatening, non-oppressive, and non-embittered way. Without the spiritual dimension, loneliness and despair creep in.

This is really the best time of life for me. I've accepted my limitations as well as my achievements. In working with younger men, I've been able to heal some of my own pain from the past. Most recently, I've begun to paint, something I never had time to do when I was younger and was so busy with work and the demands of family and friends. We turned an old garage into a nice studio where I love to work. I started taking singing lessons, for no other reason than to learn to enjoy singing more. I never felt I could carry a tune. But my teacher has been encouraging. She says, "If you can walk, you can dance. If you can talk, you can sing."

Josh's Story

I just finished reading your book *Male Menopause* and wanted to say thanks! It has helped me understand a lot. I turned sixty in July and now recognize a lot of what I had been going through.

The combination of a stressful practice, marital tensions that resulted in a divorce, and internal changes and frustrations all led to my "retirement." I was burned out. I felt lost and confused and, alone. I did what needed to be done and little else and tried to sort out what was going on inside me. It was a rough road, but I feel it has been successful.

Now, nearly seven years later, I am ecstatically married and, through my beloved's gentle and loving encouragement, I am again embarking on my career. This time it is for fun!

My wife and I have been married nearly five years now and for us, the primary commitment is to God. Like a triangle with the top point being God and each of us on the other points, we find that as we move closer to God, we move closer to each other. We also have found that through our service to others we move closer to God.

My wife is sixty and has gone through her own menopause passage. Since sex seems to be a major concern of this passage, I'd like to share what we have learned so far. Communication and consultation are vital to our lives together. We started out having "talk baths." Its hard to be less than honest when you're sitting face to face naked in the tub. Whatever was on top was the subject and the rules were simple: prayers first, then one listened carefully. Then we'd switch, still on the same topic. Then, and only then, consultation would begin with the effort being to find the "truth" and how to apply it.

After the first few years, the trust developed and the "talk baths" no longer needed to be in the tub. We have become very close as a result of these talk baths, and this has affected our sexual relationship.

Since we have a spiritual foundation in our marriage, our sexual relationship has taken on a different form. It's the bonding, the intimacy, the healing, the closeness, the expression of our love for each other, and in reality, for God, that we're after. It is the energy of creation that keeps us alive. We are learning that the physical action of intercourse is the "frosting on the cake." When the equipment works, it works, and when it doesn't, it doesn't. I'm learning that that's OK, too. The fact that we enjoy ourselves is more important.

The best part of it is that the joy of the loving energy permeates all of our activities—as long as we don't interfere with it (like focus on performance). I think we should eliminate the word "performance" from the dictionary of human relationships. I hope our experiences can be of help to others.

Gentle Men/Wild Women: Understanding the Mid-Life Gender Shift in Love, Sex, and Power

Just when I thought I'd finally gotten comfortable with what it means to be a man and what a woman really wants, things began to shift in our lives. During our years of marriage, Carlin and I had settled into a satisfying and stable routine. I had the major money-making role with a career that often took me on the road. Carlin's career brought in less money but allowed her to spend time at home with the children. We were both making our way through menopause.

After recovering from surgery, I decided that I wanted to relax more and work less. We moved to the country and to my surprise I loved the slower pace. I could spend hours splitting wood and I prided myself on spending quality time in the hammock each day. Where in the past I loved to travel, now I had no interest in exotic places. I much preferred to stay at home.

Carlin, on the other hand, was bursting with new energy. She began to expand her work in the world. She found she was becoming increasingly sought after as a counselor and spiritual mentor. She began to travel more and deepened her work with women. Even her time at home was much more demanding.

She planted a city-block-sized garden and became a farmer with tasks that needed to be accomplished each day and throughout the seasons. She watered, fertilized, weeded, planted, and harvested. She terraced the hillside and pounded in iron re-bar to shore up the boards that held her fruit trees. She put in an irrigation system which had to be monitored and cleaned periodically. She was so busy I had to remind her that we needed to take time for us. That used to be her role. Now it was me who was suggesting a day to ourselves.

It seemed to be my turn to read relationship articles and books to get clues about keeping our marriage alive and well. We seemed nearly to have reversed roles. I found a similar process going on with many of my friends and clients. Many couples become confused, and even frightened, over this shift in behavior. They long for the past when things seemed, if not more comfortable, at least more predictable. Many become lost and angry. They don't understand what's going on.

They often blame each other or blame themselves. It's not uncommon for one member of the couple to have an affair or end a marriage during this stage of life. What's going on? At first I thought it must just be our relationship. It felt like we were drifting apart and I blamed Carlin for the increasing distance between us. I wanted to feel loved and cared for. Instead, I felt neglected, like I was at the bottom of her priority list. I would alternate between being a clinging, love-sick adolescent and being an angry, demanding adolescent. Either way, I didn't feel like an adult and I hated her for making me feel that way, and I hated myself for not being able to stand tall and be the man I envisioned myself as being.

I often fantasized about finding another woman who would really want and need me and would appreciate and validate me. I really didn't want to run off and find someone else, I just wanted my wife back. She would tell me, it was my constant anger that was pushing her away. I would tell her, usually angrily, that if she would show me more love and affection, I wouldn't be so angry. We were stuck. The more I demanded, the more she withdrew. The more she withdrew, the more I demanded.

We needed to understand a whole different way of looking at our relationship in order to break the cycle of anger and withdrawal that was strangling our marriage. I came across the writings of Professor David Gutmann, author of *Reclaimed Powers*, who found that this role reversal at midlife was found in cultures throughout the world. This was validated by anthropologist Angeles Arrien. In midlife, the man seems to be drawn back toward home, back toward the center. Arrien calls this the *magnetic dimension*. The woman is driven by the opposite—*dynamic dimension*. The adventurer in her begins to assert itself, and she wants to move outward toward the periphery.

In evaluating cross-cultural data from around the world, Professor Gutmann says that a significant sex-role turnover takes place as men begin to live out directly, to own as part of themselves, the qualities of *"sensuality, affiliation, and maternal tendencies"*—in effect, the 'femininity' that was previously repressed in the service of productivity and lived out vicariously through the wife.

"By the same token, across societies," continues Gutmann, "we see the opposite effect in women. They generally become more *domineering, independent, unsentimental,* and *self-centered.*"

There is a hormonal basis for this midlife gender crossover. As estrogen levels drop for women, the testosterone/estrogen ratio increases. As testosterone levels drop for men, the estrogen/testosterone ratio increases. In fact, older men produce more estrogen and have higher levels of estrogen in their brains than post-menopausal women do. This helps account for the fact that men become gentler and more introspective while women become more outspoken and outgoing.

As my wife, Carlin, and I move through menopause, these are exactly the changes we notice in ourselves and each other. It is the source of our greatest joy and also the source of our greatest conflict. In order to keep a marriage alive and thriving during these years, we understand that we must adapt to these changes.

Many couples operate from two models of relationship for later life. One is to try and hold on to our old roles—Man: dynamic, work away, produce, protect. Woman: magnetic, work at home, provide, nurture. Or we try to shed our roles completely and take on a "unisex" model where we become elder twins. Not bad if you want to spend the rest of your life with your sister (or brother), but not very sexy.

There is a third choice that leads to health and success in marriage. I believe it is up to men to expand their masculinity and reclaim the magnetic qualities of Second Adulthood. We need to accept our "feminine" sides and be willing to enjoy our sensuality, emotionality, and romantic natures. This is the only way we will feel like real men. It won't happen by clinging to the manhood of First Adulthood. It's just not satisfying in later life. It won't happen either by trying to shed all sense of manliness, merge with our partner, and just be a "good guy." And it won't happen alone.

The truth is the newly emerging "magnetic man" will be eaten alive by the newly emerging "dynamic woman," unless he gets a great deal of support from the community of men.

I've found that women today have little sympathy for simpering men who can't find their masculinity and hope women will take care of them. An elder woman's mothering instincts can still be tapped when their grown children (or grandchildren) are in danger, when their friends need help, or when the community needs a fierce protector. But with their husbands and lovers they do indeed tend to exhibit their older-woman dynamism that researcher David Gutmann found to be true across the globe: domineering, independent, unsentimental, and self-centered.

It's the reason I have been in a men's group for the past twenty years and intend to be in one the rest of my life. It's the only way that is possible for me to match the energy of the older woman in my life. If we are going to be equals, I have found, I need a continual renewal of male care and support that I can only get when I am in the presence of other men.

It's the reason you see elder males in traditional cultures hanging out with their peers—telling jokes, having fun, eating, drinking, singing, dancing, telling stories, embracing each other, talking about their last sexual encounter, and planning their next. Men today have a lot to learn from these traditional cultures with their ancient practices which have been honed for thousands of years.

I have found there are ten key issues a man must engage if he is to be successful in the second half of life.

1. Recognize That Male Menopause is a Preparation Stage for Super Adulthood

Think what it would be like if we could skip puberty and go directly to being adults. We could avoid all those nasty physical changes in our bodies—no skin blemishes, no pimples. We wouldn't have all the teenage akwardness, mood swings, and emotional volatility. Our hormones wouldn't whip through us like storms on the sea. We wouldn't worry about first sexual experiences, venereal disease, or teen pregnancy. We could avoid thinking about whether to go to college, take time traveling, or get a job, whether to invest in a car, or save for the future.

But we wouldn't get to practice being an adult. We would be thrust into it. Could you imagine going from being a smooth-skinned, emotionally stable, ten-year-old living at home with Mom and Dad, to being a twenty-five-year-old, newly married adult moving into your first condo? We might avoid some of the growing pains of adolescence, but we would lose the transition period that prepares us to be adults. Similarly with male menopause, we need these fifteen or so years of disruption and turmoil to allow us to prepare for the next stage of our lives—super-adulthood.

2. Let Go of Old Patterns and Heal Past Traumas

This is a time to change our way of looking at ourselves and the world, to break free of old patterns and heal old wounds.

While Carlin and I were talking over breakfast the other day, I told her about a dream I had the previous night. In the dream I was being asked to marry a younger woman. I didn't really want to do this, but for some reason I felt compelled to go through with the marriage. I thought at least I will enjoy having sex with a younger woman. On the day of the wedding, I decided I couldn't go through with it. I loved Carlin and wanted to stay married to her.

When we analyzed the dream together, I said that the young woman in the dream represented my adolescent self, the "Jewish American Prince" that feels he is entitled to have what he wants when he wants it. I felt that Carlin in the dream represented the part of me that gives to others, is mature and cares about himself, works hard, and doesn't demand or whine.

Carlin laughed and said, "Sounds like you're choosing to grow up." I laughed too. "Yeah, I guess it does."

This is often a time where we must go back into our past and deal with unfinished business. We come to terms with things we didn't get from our parents, dreams that we didn't achieve. We also learn to appreciate what we did get and what we have accomplished.

We behave less like victims and more like self-directed adults. We feel more joy and gratitude for life and are more accepting of ourselves and others. We forgive ourselves for the hurt we have caused others and forgive those who we believe have hurt us.

3. Move from the Pressure of Sexual Performance to the Joy of Sexual Fulfillment

Our early sexual encounters were fraught with uncertainty and excitement. For most of us, we come to terms with our sexual selves and things perk along through adulthood until we hit male menopause and it feels like we are losing all the ease and confidence we have gained. As our testosterone falls, so does our sexual desire, self-confidence, our sense of male pride, and our sexual stamina.

But don't be too eager to find something that will allow you to perform like you did when you were young. This is a time when we can be relieved of the whole burden of performance all together. Sex can become a means of celebrating our togetherness, not just a vehicle for achieving an orgasm. It can be full-bodied, robust, and playful when it doesn't have to perform for anyone. Sex can be fun again.

4. Focus More on Being and Less on Doing

During our adult years, there is a great deal of focus on doing things. We do our school assignments. We do our work. We do the dishes. We do the bills. We do the car repairs. We do the housework. We may slip into becoming human-doings and lose the sense that we are human-beings. But this is the time of life that we have more opportunity just to be.

I remember as a young adult feeling the responsibilities of finding a job, getting married, having children, raising children, keeping the money coming in to buy the things my wife and children needed.

I worried a lot about failing, but I kept on going and kept on going and kept on going. It was like a race I felt I had to win. One day, I realized that I had already crossed the finish line and I didn't even know it. All five children were grown and on their own. My wife had her own work and was quite capable of taking care of herself.

I realized I could sit back and enjoy more time just being alive. I could be with my family. I could be with my friends. I could be awake all night if I wanted to and I could be asleep until noon if it pleased me. I could be giving when I felt like it and be selfish when I wanted to give to myself. I could be my own boss, work for someone else, or take time and not work at all. I could be an artist or a poet or just be a guy who sits on his back porch and watches the day go by. Most of all, I could just be alive and thank my lucky stars that so much love has come my way in my life.

5. Change from Having a Career Based on Necessity to a Calling Based on Soul-Work

Most of us start our adult lives taking a job out of necessity. We have to eat. We need to pay for shelter. We have responsibilities we feel we must meet. Sometimes one job leads to another and we get locked into a career, not because it is what we love to do, but because we feel we need to do it. If we are lucky we are able to hold on to our jobs and raise our families. If we are not lucky we are displaced before we are ready. Our business is downsized and we have to hit the pavement and find another job.

At this time of life, we have a choice. We can begin to ask ourselves what we love, what we would do even if we didn't get paid for doing it. We can ask what our soul calling might be. I have a good friend who quit his job of twenty years as vice president of a bank to go into business for himself as a consultant. I have another friend who retired from his work as director of a large social service agency to pursue his dream to be a painter. Another friend retired from being a counselor and returned to his love, playing violin.

I cut back on my work as a writer, consultant, and therapist to learn to do flamenco dancing and to work with high school student counselors.

This is a time to pursue our dreams and allow ourselves to give our gifts to ourselves, our families, friends, and community.

6. Relate to Other Men as Friends and Allies Rather than Competitors

I still remember when I started my first men's group nearly twenty-five years ago. We all felt a need for contact with other men, but we were also reluctant to open up and share our most personal experiences. Our experiences with other men in the past had taught us to be wary of men. We all worried, though we didn't voice our concern, that letting men know our weaknesses would put us at a disadvantage.

We were sure that if another man had a chance he would move in on the woman in our life or try and take our job. Though we could be friends with other guys, we saw them as competitors. If there was a choice, we were sure, we'd bet the other guy would sell out our friendship if he could get something he wanted.

I still remember the first time the thought was tested. Gary had been seeing Sue but Bob had a liking for her as well. At one meeting, Gary finally voiced his concern that Bob would try and take her away if he had a chance. I still remember Bob's reply, "I couldn't do that, Gary." His voice showed he meant it. "Your friendship means more to me than winning a woman."

It was a breakthrough for the group. We realized we had been wrong about each other. As we had gotten older, friendship mattered more. We found we were supporting each others' relationships, sharing our joy when a man got a job promotion, and helping each other when we felt stuck. It's wonderful to feel that kind of security that allows us to open up, share our vulnerabilities, and allow friendships to grow.

7. End the Battle of the Sexes and Find Intimacy, Passion, and Joy with Your Life Partner

Before I turned fifty, I thought that there was something about men and women that inevitably brought them into conflict. My whole adult life seemed to be a roller coaster when I was with a woman. Mostly things were up, but when they were down the pain was excruciating.

Looking back, I realized that I still felt wounded by past relationships. Even though I put up a strong front at the time, I was deeply hurt. I used the old hurts and fears of abandonment as a shield, an attempt to protect myself from having it happen again. As a result, I never felt totally comfortable with my wife. I knew she could hurt me more than anyone else could.

However, as we both passed the fifty mark and moved into the next phase of our relationship, things began to shift. We made a conscious choice to live our lives from the assumption of love and good will rather than from anger and fear. If there was some disagreement with Carlin that in the past I would interpret as her desire to hurt me, I now saw it as a loving gesture that had gone awry.

I felt stronger and more secure with myself and less in need of proving myself right. We could laugh and joke about our many foibles and failings without blaming the other person. I was amazed at the different quality of the love that was expressed when we no longer needed to be prepared for battle on a moment's notice.

Intimacy, passion, and joy only can grow in an atmosphere of compassion and goodwill. These are qualities I could call on only intermittently in my early years. It's wonderful, as I get older, to feel them more present in my life and in my relationship on an ongoing basis.

8. Become a Mentor to Young Men and Women

I've been blessed with five children in my life, my son and daughter with my first wife and three sons that Carlin brought into my life when she and I got together. I had always been a father to my son and daughter and gradually became a father figure to Carlin's sons.

But whether we have children or not, the second half of life is a time when we feel drawn to being a mentor to the next generation. Often, we aren't even aware we are doing anything special. Carlin and I are involved in a small theater group in our community. In one of the productions I worked with a number of teenagers in the community. I would often see one of the girls in town and would stop and ask her how she was doing. We would chat for a few minutes and be on our way.

I didn't think much of it. I was just being friendly and caring. I was genuinely interested in how things were going for her. Two years later, I was working with teens in the high school. The girl from the theater also was involved in the teen program. In one of the support groups, she told me with tears in her eyes how much it meant to her that I kept a connection. "I always liked seeing you," she told me. "I felt like you cared about how my life was going and kind of kept track of me as I was getting older." It brought tears to my own eyes knowing that with such a simple gesture I was making a difference in her life.

In the high school program, I have had an opportunity to counsel some of the boys as well. I've found it is so important to have a male figure who is not part of their family who believes in them and can encourage them.

But whatever I have been able to contribute to the lives of youngsters has been overshadowed by what they have contributed to me. Being able to feel that my life experience counts for something, that there are things I have to offer younger men and women in my community, knowing that I make a difference in the lives of these people, makes me feel alive and worthwhile.

I don't think we can feel complete as men in the second half of our lives unless we find a way we can contribute to those who will be living after we are gone. It is particularly important that we provide support for young men. Without the caring guidance of older men, the aggressive energy of young men often turns to senseless violence.

9. Learn What It Takes to Be a Respected Elder in Your Community

In a society like ours where so many older men and women become obsessed with the desire to look and feel young, we pay too little attention to the importance of becoming a respected elder.

One of my teachers, Malidoma Some, comes from a traditional tribal community in Africa. He has made me aware of the vital importance of this role in any society if we are to survive and prosper. "Elders and mentors have an irreplaceable function in the life of any community," he says. "Without them, the young are lost—their overflowing energies wasted in useless pursuits. The old must live in the young like a grounding force that tames the tendency towards bold but senseless actions and shows them the path of wisdom. In the absence of elders, the impetuosity of youth becomes the slow death of the community."

The importance of eldering, both for the man himself and for the society, seems to be universal. In traditional societies throughout Africa, for example, one of the prime roles of older men is as "Peacemaker." Anthropologist Paul Spencer found this role is prevalent among the Samburu of East Africa (an offshoot tribe of the bellicose Masai), as well as the Zulu, the Nyakyusa, and the Lele of Central Africa. They recognize that the young men must express their aggression, but they also recognize that the role of elder males is to channel and control it.

In our society, we either deny the aggression of young men or punish it by locking them up. Neither approach works well—we continue to see an increasing level of violence in our society while our prisons fill up with young males who never had the support of the elders in their communities.

Says Professor David Gutmann, who has written extensively about these traditional societies, "While the old men of these tribes might recognize that the intemperate young man is the best vessel for the collective aggression of the group, they also recognize that this aggression must be physically removed from the vulnerable precincts of the intimate community."

In studying other indigenous cultures, two other roles arise as important for men. Elder males, in addition to their role in keeping order in the community, attend to the community's *spiritual* needs and provide *mentoring* for the young males.

All three of these roles—Peacemaker, Spirit Guide, and Mentor—are as important to our culture as they are to indigenous societies. They offer older men specific roles for their later years. They offer young men the kind of support they need to channel their youthful aggression into constructive channels. They offer the members of the larger society the kind of protection they need to feel safe and secure.

10. Be a Trailblazer for Experiencing a Life Well Lived into Your Seventies, Eighties, Nineties, and Beyond

Carlin and I just got back from visiting our neighbors Mary and Al. Both are in their mid-eighties and both maintain an active life. Al retired at sixty-five after a lifetime of hard work, and he and Mary moved to Arizona to relax and enjoy their senior years. As happens to many who retire, they thought they'd kick back and relax in their retirement, but instead, they got old, sick, and bored. Their daughter invited them to move to California and they now live in a small trailer behind their daughter's house.

Mary continued with the things she loved—cooking, baking, sewing, talking to family and friends. Al found a new lease on life. He began working outside, cutting wood, planting a garden, doing repairs. He lost his pot belly and found that he wasn't ready to retire. When his granddaughter bought him a computer, his life was transformed. He learned to use it, got on the Internet, and now is developing a number of home-based businesses.

"What's the difference between these businesses and all the other ones you've tried that didn't work," Mary wanted to know. Al smiled and patted his computer. "I never had the support of a worldwide network of potential customers before." He's having the time of his life he says…and it shows. Whenever we visit, he always has time to listen to me and give advice on what I can do to expand my work. Most mornings, when I turn on my computer there is a note from Al with some new and interesting findings from the Web.

Al isn't the only one who has "retired from retirement" and is enjoying a full and rewarding life on the Second Mountain. A new survey found that new challenges and adventures, rather than old-fashioned ideas of rest and more rest stretching into an indefinite future are what more and more elders are looking forward to having.

The survey showed that only 32 percent of the retirees and 23 percent of those close to it viewed retirement as "a time to take it easy, take care of yourself, enjoy leisure activities, and take a much-deserved rest from work and daily responsibilities."

But at the opposite end of the question, 61 percent of the retirees and 70 percent of non-retirees saw it as "a time to begin a new chapter." That attitude appeared to be reflected in other reports and surveys showing that older men and women—not only in America, but also in Europe and the rest of the world—are increasingly involved in skiing, trekking, and other activities that for long had been considered activities exclusive to the young.

And why not have some of both. As we live longer and healthier lives, there will be time for relaxation and enjoyment, as well as the excitement of new adventures. "I'm having more fun than I've ever had," Al tells me. "I can't wait to get up in the morning and get started. Life is good."

As I end this book, I think of two important elders in my life. My father who lived to be ninety taught me the joy of being involved in life from beginning to end. My friend and mentor, Sidney, who is in his late eighties and is still going strong, continues to teach me that exercise, good food, and a sexually active and loving relationship are the cornerstones of a life well-lived.

Let Me Hear From You

Your letters have been heartening. I am busy working on another book. I would very much like to hear from your experiences of what has worked for you, what hasn't worked, and what information you'd like to know more about. If you are a health care professional that works with male menopause, let me know. I am continually being asked for referrals. I read all my letters personally and look forward to hearing from you.

Send letters to:

Jed Diamond

MenAlive

34133 Shimmins Ridge Rd.

Willits, CA 95490

Email: Jed@MenAlive.com

website: www.MenAlive.com

Bibliography

Barash, David P., and Judith Eve Lipton, M.D. *Making Sense of Sex: How Genes and Gender Influence Our Relationships.* Washington, D.C.: Island Press, 1997.

Benson, Herbert, and Marg Stark. *Timeless Healing: The Power and Biology of Belief.* New York: Scribner, 1996.

Blankenhorn, David. *Fatherless America: Confronting Our Most Urgent Social Problem.* New York: Basic Books, 1995.

Bly, Robert. *Iron John: A Book About Men.* New York: Addison-Wesley, 1990.

————. *The Sibling Society.* New York: Addison-Wesley, 1996.

Bortz, Walter M. *Dare to Be 100.* New York: Fireside, 1996.

Borysenko, Joan. *Minding the Body, Mending the Mind.* New York: Addison-Wesley, 1987.

———. *A Woman's Book of Life: The Biology, Psychology and Sprituality of the Feminine Life Cycle.* New York: Riverhead Books, 1996.

Buss, David M. *The Evolution of Desire: Strategies of Human Mating.* New York: Basic Books, 1994.

Carruthers, Malcolm, M.D. *Maximizing Manhood: Beating The Male Menopause.* London: HarperCollins, 1997.

Clark, Etta. *Growing Old Is Not for Sissies: Portraits of Senior Athletes.* Corte Madera, Calif.: Pomegranate Calendars and Books, 1986.

Coney, Sandra. *The Menopause Industry: How the Medical Establishment Exploits Women.* Alameda, Calif.: Hunter House, 1994.

Cowley, Geoffrey. "Attention Aging Men: Testosterone and Other Hormone Treatments Offer New Hope for Staying Youthful, Sexy and Strong." *Newsweek* 16 Sept. 1996: 68+.

———. "My Month on DHEA: One Man's Experiment with Hormone Therapy." *Newsweek* 16 Sept. 1996: 74.

Crenshaw, Theresa. *The Alchemy of Love and Lust: Discovering Our Sex Hormones and How They Determine Who We Love, When We Love, and How Often We Love.* New York: G.P. Putnam's Sons, 1996.

Cutler, Winnifred B. *Love Cycles: The Science of Intimacy.* New York: Villard Books, 1991.

Diamond, Jed. *Male Menopause.* Naperville, Ill.: Sourcebooks, 1997, 1998.

———. *The Warrior's Journey Home: Healing Men, Healing the Planet.* Oakland, Calif.: New Harbinger Publications, 1994.

Fisher, Helen. *The First Sex: The Natural Talents of Women and How They Are Changing The World.* New York: Random House, 1999.

———. *Anatomy of Love: The Mysteries of Mating, Marriage, and Why We Stray.* New York: Ballantine Books, 1992.

Gillette, Douglas M. *Primal Love: Reclaiming Our Instincts for Lasting Passion*. New York: St. Martin's Press, 1995.

Goldberg, Ken. *How Men Can Live as Long as Women: Seven Steps to a Longer and Better Life*. Fort Worth: The Summit Group, 1993.

Gottman, John., and Nan Silver. *The Seven Principles For Making Marriage Work*. New York: Crown Publishers, 1999.

Gottman, John. *Why Marriages Succeed or Fail*. New York: Simon & Schuster, 1994.

Green, James. *The Male Herbal: Health Care for Men and Boys*. Freedom, Calif.: The Crossing Press, 1991.

Gurian, Michael. *The Wonder of Boys: What Parents, Mentors and Educators Can Do to Shape Boys into Exceptional Men*. New York: G.P. Putnam's Sons, 1996.

Gutmann, David. *Reclaimed Powers: Men and Women in Later Life*. Evanston, Ill.: Northwestern University Press, 1994.

Hallowell, Edward M., M.D. *Worry: Controlling It and Using It Wisely*. New York: Pantheon Books, 1997.

Hallowell, Edward M., M.D. and John J. Rately, M.D. *Driven to Distraction: Recognizing and Coping With Attention Deficit Disorder From Childhood Through Adulthood*. New York: Touchstone, 1995.

Hayflick, Leonard. *How and Why We Age*. New York: Ballantine Books, 1994.

Hill, Aubrey M. *Viropause/Andropause: The Male Menopause: Emotional and Physical Changes Mid-Life Men Experience*. Far Hills, N.J.: New Horizon Press, 1993.

———. *Testosterone: New Ways to Revitalize Your Life with Male Hormone Therapy*. Sacramento, Calif.: Prima Publishing, 1997.

Janeway, Elizabeth. *Man's World, Woman's Place: A Study In Social Mythology*. New York: Dell, 1971.

Jones, Dan. *What Makes a Man a Man*. Austin, Texas: Mandala Books, 1993.

Levinson, Daniel J. *The Seasons of a Man's Life*. New York: Ballantine Books, 1978.

————. *The Seasons of a Woman's Life*. New York: Alfred A. Knopf, 1996.

Michael, Robert T., John H. Gagnon, Edward O. Laumann, and Gina Kolata. *Sex in America: A Definitive Survey*. New York: Warner Books, 1994.

Miedzian, Myriam. *Boys Will Be Boys: Breaking the Link Between Masculinity and Violence*. New York: Doubleday, 1991.

Miller, Alice. *For Your Own Good: Hidden Cruelty in Child Rearing and the Roots of Violence*. New York: Farrar, Strauss, & Giroux, 1983.

Miller, Timothy. *How to Want What You Have: Discovering the Magic and Grandeur of Ordinary Existence*. New York: Avon Books, 1995.

Official Journal of the International Society for the Study of The Aging Male. "The Aging Male." London: The Parthenon Publishing Group.

Paley, Maggie. *The Book of The Penis*. New York: Grove Press, 1999.

Pearsall, Paul. *Sexual Healing: Using the Power of an Intimate, Loving Relationship to Heal Your Body and Soul*. New York: Crown Publishers, Inc., 1994.

Rako, Susan. *The Hormone of Desire*. New York: Harmony Books, 1996.

Real, Terrence. *I Don't Want to Talk About It: Overcoming the Secrecy of Male Depression*. New York: Scribner, 1997.

Regelson, William, M.D., and Carol Coleman. *The Superhomone Promise: Nature's Antidote to Aging*. New York: Simon & Schuster, 1996.

Reitz, Rosetta. *Menopause: A Positive Approach*. New York: Chilton Book Co., 1977.

Roth, Dick. *No, It's Not Hot In Here—A Husband's Guide to Understanding Menopause.* Georgetown, Mass.: Ant Hill Press, 1999.

Schneider, Jennifer, and Burt Schneider. *Sex, Lies, and Forgiveness: Couples Speaking Out on Healing From Sex Addiction.* Center City, Minn.: Hazelden, 1991.

Segell, Michael. "The New Softness. (Why Men Become More Intimate and Nurturing in Later Life)." *Esquire* April 1996: 51.

Sheehy, Gail. *New Passages: Mapping Your Life Across Time.* New York: Random House, 1995.

Shippen, Eugene, M.D., and William Fryer. *The Testosterone Syndrome: The Critical Factor For Energy, Health, and Sexuality—Reversing The Male Menopause.* New York: M. Evans and Company, 1998.

Small, Meredith F. *What's Love Got to Do with It? The Evolution of Human Mating.* New York: Doubleday, 1995.

Tannen, Deborah. *You Just Don't Understand: Women and Men in Conversation.* New York: Ballantine Books, 1990.

Vanzant, Iyanla. *The Spirit of a Man: A Vision of Transformation for Black Men and the Women Who Love Them.* New York: Harper Collins, 1996.

Walsh, Patrick C., and Janet Farrar Worthington. *The Prostate: A Guide for Men and the Women Who Love Them.* Baltimore: Johns Hopkins University Press, 1995.

Wright, Jonathan V., M.D., and Lane Lenard. *Maximize Your Vitality and Potency: For Men Over 40.* Petaluma, Calif.: Smart Publications, 1999.

Resources

Aging

The International Society For the Study of the Aging Male
The Parthenon Publishing Group
Casterton Hall, Carnforth
Lancs LA6 2LA, UK
Tel: 44(0) 15242 72084
Fax: 44(0) 15242 71587
Email: mail@parthpub.com
This organization is dedicated to improving the health status, longevity, and quality of life of the aging male. They publish the journal, *The Aging Male*, and sponsor professional conferences.

National Institute on Aging
800-222-2225 (8:30 –5 EST)

AIDS

Naitonal CDC HIV/AIDS Hotline
800-342-2437 (24-hour hotline)

Alternative Medicine

Office of Alternative Medicine
U.S. Government
9000 Rockville Pike
Boilding 51, Room 5B-37
Mailstop 2181
Betheseda, MD 29892
888-644-6226 (8:30–5 EST)

American Holistic Medical Association
4101 Lake Boon Trail, Suite 201
Raleigh, NC 27607

Physicians Committee for Responsible Medicine
5100 Wisconsin Ave NW, Suite 404
Washington, DC 20016
202-686-2210

Alzheimer's Disease

Alzheimer's Association
800-272-3900 (8–5 CST)

Arthritis

Arthritis Foundation
800-283-7800 (24-hour recording)

Attention Deficit Disorder

Daniel F. Amen, M.D.
350 Chadbourne Rd.
Fairfield, CA 94585
707-429-7181
www.amenclinic.com
Extensive information on Attention Deficit Disorder (ADD) in adults, teens, and children. Website has links to a great deal of information in the field.

Cancer

American Cancer Society
800-227-2345 (24-hour recording)

Career Management

The Venture Hill Project's Career Management Group
P.O. Box 9568
Santa Rosa, CA 95405-1568
Email: hlagarde@wco.com
Developed by Howard LaGarde, this project operates from a context of "Lives Well Lived" and supports men and women in developing careers that balance personal, interpersonal, and planetary needs.

Drugs/Alcohol

National Clearinghouse for Alcohol and Drug Information
800-729-6686 (8–7 EST)

Ecology and Cultural Renewal

Museletter
Richard Heinberg
1433 Olivet Rd.
Santa Rosa, CA 95401
www.museletter.com/museletter/
Email: rheinberg@igc.org
A wonderful monthly newsletter that explores the roots of our heritage back to hunter/gatherer times and offers hopeful alternatives for the future.

Ecopsychology Institute
California State University, Hayward
25800 Carlos Bee Blvd.
Hayward, CA 94542-3045
510-885-3236
Email: ecopsy@csuhayward.edu

Environment and Health

Environmental Health Clearinghouse
800-643-4794 (9–8 EST)

Eyes

National Eye Institute
301-496-5248 (8:30–5 EST)

Grandparenting

Foundation for Grandparenting
5 Casa del Oro Lane
Santa Fe, NM 87505

Hearing

National Institute on Deafness and Other Communication
Disorders
800-241-1044 (8:30–5 EST)

Heart

American Heart Association
800-AHA-USA1 (8:30–4:30 local time)

Herbal Information

California School of Herbal Studies
James Green and James Snow Codirectors
P.O. Box 39
Forestville, CA 95436
707-887-7457

James Green, who is the author or *The Male Herbal*, also has written
the *Herbal Medicine-Makers Handbook*.

Incontinence

The Simon Foundation for Continence
800-237-4666 (24-hours)

Longevity and Health

American Academy of Anti-Aging Medicine
401 North Michigan Ave.
Chicago, IL 60611-6610

Life Enhancement

P.O. Box 751390

Petaluma, CA 94975-9846

800-543-3873

707-762-6144

Fax 707-769-8016

Life Enhancement offers nutritional supplement products for slowing the aging process, enhancing cognition, increasing libido, and extending lifespan. They have been the pioneers in bringing to market DHEA, melatonin, 5-hydroxy-tryptophan, and pregnenolone. They publish a monthly newsmagazine with thoroughly researched articles on enhancing your life and better living through biochemistry.

Longevity Institute International

89 Valley Rd.

Montclair, NJ 07042

201-746-3533

Fax 201-746-4385

Lung

American Lung Association

800-LUNG-USA (9–4 EST)

Medication

Center for Drug Evaluation and Research

301-594-1012 (8:30–4:30 EST)

Men's Health

Malcolm Carruthers, M.D.
Gold Cross Medical Clinic
20/20 Harmont House
20 Harley St.
London, W1N 1AL, England
Tel: 44(0) 171 636 8283
Fax: 44 (0) 171 636 8292
www.goldcrossmedical.com
Broad information on men's health, including hormone replacement therapies. Dr. Carruthers does a complete evaluation to test for male menopause and links in with doctors in the U.S. and around the world.

Jed Diamond Presents
34133 Shimmins Ridge Rd.
Willits, CA 95490
Email: jed@menalive.com
Information on other books, booklets, tapes, seminars, and trainings by Jed Diamond; updated information on male menopause and men; listing of physicians and other health professionals who specialize in working with men going through the male menopause passage. (If you are a professional and wish to be listed, send a description of your practice.)

The Male Health Center
Kenneth A Goldberg, M.D.
5744 LBJ Freeway, Suite 100
Dallas, TX 75240
972-420-8500

Men's Health Network
Ronald K Henry, Esq., Director
310 D Street NE
Washington, DC 20002
202-543-6461
Email: mensnet@capaccess.org

Men's Healthline
888-636-2636
(Toll-free number for health information specific to men)

TotalCare Medical Center
Alan P. Brauer, M.D.
630 University Ave.
Palo Alto, CA 94301
415-329-8001

Jonathan V. Wright, M.D.
Medical Director
Tahoma Clinic
515 W. Harrison St.
Kent, Washington 98032
253-854-4900
Fax: 253-850-5639
www.tahoma-clinic.com

Men's Initiation and Mentoring

New Warrior Network
Drury Heffernan
Box 230
Malone, NY 12953-0230
Email: dhnwmtl@aol.com
An order of men called to reclaim the sacred masculine for our time, through initiation, training, and action in the world.

Sterling Institute of Relationship
695 Rand Ave.
Oakland, CA 94610
510-836-1400
Dedicated to transforming the quality of people's relationships to produce the partnership and the context necessary for the transition to a true global community.

Men's Issues

Men's Rights, Inc. (MR, Inc.)
Fred Hayward, Executive Director
Box 163180
Sacramento, CA 95816
916-484-7333
A nonprofit corporation that raises public awareness about all men's issues. Their egalitarian philosophy is: equal rights for men and women...no exceptions.

National Organization of Circumcision Information Resource Centers
P.O. Box 2512
San Anselmo, CA 94979-2512
415-488-9883
Provides the most accurate and up-to-date information on the effects of circumcision on males. Sponsors international conferences on both male and female circumcision worldwide.

National Organization to Halt the Abuse and Routine Mutilation of Males (NOHARMM)
P.O. Box 460795
San Francisco, CA 94146
415-826-9351
A national, non-violent direct-action network of men organized against routine infant circumcision.

Men/Fathers Hotline

512-472-3237

A crisis line for men and their fathers.

Wingspan: Journal of the Male Spirit

P.O. Box 265

North Lake, WI 53064

619-454-4622

Fax 619-454-4851

Email: honeycreek@aol.com

An international quarterly journal with wide-ranging focus on various aspects of the men's movement.

Men's Resources on the Web—General Information

MenWeb

www.vix.com/menmag/

MenWeb features interviews with bestselling authors, insightful articles, men's stories, poems, and a wealth of information on men's growth and personal development. Website for *Men's Voices*, successor to *M.E.N. Magazine*, the content is wide-ranging but also has a "men's movement" and Jungian focus. Areas on fathers, relationships, fathering, men's groups, and other topics.

Men's Issues Page

www.vix.com/pub/men/index.html

An encyclopedic index of men's issues resources. The most complete index and archive of men's articles, issues, organizations, books, and resources.

Menstuff, The National Men's Resource

www.menstuff.org/

A calendar listing international, national, and regional men's conferences, workshops, and gatherings.

The Men's Resource Network

www.TheMensCenter.com

The internet portal to the wide world of men. A tremendous gathering of current men's groups and organizations as well as listing of resources.

Manhood Online (Australia)

www.manhood.com.av/

This site centers on the work of Steve Biddulph, author of Australian bestseller *Manhood*. Their "Manzine" has lots of interesting articles. The site also serves as a coordinating point for Men's Work around Australia. A calendar listing national and regional men's events and resource catalog round out the offerings.

Crisis, Grief, and Healing: Men and Women

www.webhealing.com

This is a place men and women can browse to understand and honor the many different paths to heal strong emotions. It has a special emphasis on how men often grieve differently. Tom Golden, LCSW of Washington, C.D., is and internationally known psychotherapist, author, and speaker on the topic of healing from loss.

M.A.L.E.: Men Assisting, Leading, and Educating

www.malesurvivor.org/

M.A.L.E is dedicated to helping male survivors of sexual abuse to heal.

Vietnam Veterans Page

http://www.vietvet.org/index.htm

This is an interactive online forum for Vietnam veterans and their families and friends to exchange information, stories, poems, songs, art, pictures, and experiences in any publishing form.

Men's Resources on the Web—Health Information

[sub]The Male Health Center

http://www.malehealthcenter.com

The Male Health Center in Dallas, Texas, founded by Dr. Ken Goldberg has an excellent website on important aspects of male health.

North American Menopause Society

http://www.menopause.com

Current research information on menopause.

CaP CURE: The Association for the Cure of Cancer of Prostate

http://www.capcure.org/

The Association for the Cure of Cancer of the Prostate, CaP CURE, is a non profit public charity dedicated to finding a cure for prostate cancer by rapidly funding promising basic and clinical research.

Prostatitis Home Page

www.prostatitis.org

An excellent resource concerning prostatitis and other problem problems associated with prostate gland, sponsored by the Prostatitis Foundation.

University of Michigan Prostate Cancer Home Page

http://www.cancer.med.umich.edu/prostcan/prostcan.html

A professional prostate cancer resource page.

Conditions Men Get, Too (US FDA Page)

http://www.fda.gov/fdac/features/695_men.html

Describes how men are affected by osteoporosis, breast cancer, and eating disorders—diseases traditionally thought of as "women's diseases."

Circumcision Information and Resource Pages
http://www.cirp.org/CIRP/
The Circumcision Information and Resource Pages provide information about all aspects of the genital surgery known as circumcision. The Circumcision Reference Library contains technical material, medical and historical articles, and statistics. The Circumcision Information Pages contain a more readable collection of information, suitable for parents and educators. The site also has links to information on the rights of the child, religious issues, and related issues.

Men's Resources on the Web—Fathering Information

National Center for Fathering
http://www.fathers.com/
Today's Father magazine provides an online presence and a wealth of tips and information on fathering. The mission of the National Center for Fathering is to inspire men to be better fathers and to develop practical resources to prepare dads for nearly every fathering situation.

The Divorce Page
http://hughson.com/
Dean Hughson has put together an excellent Web page on the emotional, practical, and legal problems that come up for men in divorce. It also has practical advice (e.g. how to sleep, eating well, cheap airline tickets to see the kids) and many valuable links.

United Fathers Forum
http://www.enol.com/~uff/uff.htm
Information on legislation and resources related to fathers' rights.

Men's Resources on the Web—Men's Organizations

Men's Rights, Inc.
http://www.mens-rights.org/
Men's Rights, Inc. was founded by Fredric Hayward. It sponsors a Men's Rights ERA Project, "Equal rights for men and women…no exceptions," headed by Dave Ault in Seattle.

National Coalition of Free Men
http://www.ncfm.org/
The National Coalition of Free Men (NCFM) is a nonprofit educational organization that examines that way sex discrimination affects men. It also tries to raise public consciousness about little-known, but important topics dealing with the male experience. In addition NCFM sponsors a variety of "men's rights" projects.

New Warrior Network
http://www.nwn.org
New Warrior offers opportunities for men to experience male initiation so that they can become mentors to younger men.

Menopause

Menopause Access Hotline
1-800-222-4767 (For Information)

Mental Health

Grief Recovery Helpline
1-800-445-4808 (9-5 PST)

National Institute of Mental Health
301-443-4513 (8:30-4:30 EST)

Mind/Body Healing

Mind/Body Medical Institute
110 Francis Street
Boston, MA 02215 617-632-9525
Founded and directed by Herbert Benson, M.D., the Institute offers information and resources on mind/ body healing.

Neurological Disorders

National Institute of Neurological Disorders and Stroke
301-496-5751 (8:30-5 EST)

Nutrition and Health

American Dietetic Association Nutrition Hotline
1-800-366-1655 (experts: 9-4 CST; recordings: 8-8 CST)

EarthSave
Box 68
Santa Cruz, CA 95062
831-423-4069
Founded by John Robbins, EarthSave promotes the benefits of plant-based food choices for optimal health, environmental preservation, and a more compassionate world.

Osteoporosis

National Osteoporosis Foundation
202-223-2226 (8:30-5:30 EST)

Parenting

National Institute of Child Health and Human Development
301-496-5133 (8-5 EST)

Pheromones

Athena Institute for Women's Wellness
Winnifred Cutler, Ph.D., President
610-827-2200

PMS (Pre-Menstrual Syndrome)

PMS Access
1-800-222-4767 (For further information)
1-800-558-7046 (For referrals to physicians in your area 9-5 CST)

Prostate

The Prostatitis Foundation
The nonprofit group, formed by men frustrated with their treatment, has been lobbying Congress, organizing researchers, and disseminating information. The foundation offers the following resources:
Prostatitis Information Packet. For $2, you will receive a packet of information, including a lab-test worksheet that is very helpful in getting a proper diagnosis. Foundation Membership. For $25 tax-deductible donation, you will receive a year of research updates. Write To:
The Prostatitis Foundation
Information Distribution Center
Parkway Business Center, 2929 Ireland Grove Rd.
Bloomington, IL 61704
Internet Newsgroup. You can join a supportive group of men exchanging the latest information on prostatitis by subscribing to sci.men.prostate.prostatitis.
Us-Too International
1010 Jorie Blvd., Suite 124
Oak Brook, IL 60521
1-800-808-7866
This prostate-cancer support network boasts more than 440 groups throughout America.

National Prostate Cancer Coalition, Inc.
3709 W. Jetton Avenue
Tampa, FL 33629

Rare Diseases

National Organization for Rare Disorders
1-800-999-6673 (9-5 EST; 24-hour recording)

Stroke

American Heart Association Stroke Connection
1-800-553-6321 (8:30-5 CST)
Urologic Disorders

American Foundation for Urologic Disease
300 W. Pratt St., Suite 401
Baltimore, MD 21201
410-468-1800 (8:30-5 EST)

Wellness

Ardell Wellness Report
Don Ardell, Ph.D., Publisher
9901 Lake Georgia Dr.
Orlando, FL 32817
407-657-2846

Women's Health

MidLife Women's Network
5129 Logan Ave. S
Minneapolis, MN 55419-1019
1-800-886-4354

Mind/Body Health Sciences, Inc.
Joan Borysenko, M.D., Director
393 Dixon Rd.
Boulder, Co 80302
303-440-8460

Dr. Christiane Northrup's Health Wisdom for Women Newsletter
Philips Publishing, Inc.
7811 Montrose Rd.
Potomac, MD 20897-5924
1-800-804-0935

Women's Health Advocate Newsletter
PO Box 420235
Palm Coast, FL 32132-0235
1-800-829-5876

Women's International Pharmacy
Wallace L. Simons, R.Ph., Director
Natural hormone therapy by prescription only.
1-800-279-5708

Women's Health Watch
164 Longwood Ave.
Boston, MA 02115
1-800-829-5921
A newsletter of information for enlightened choices from the Harvard Medical School.

Please let us know if there are changes we need to make in this list or other resources that should be added in future editions.
Send to:
Jed Diamond
Email: jed@menalive.com
34133 Shimmins Ridge Rd.
Willits, CA 95490

Index

life expectancy, 6
Lindsay, Robert, 77
Lipton, Judith Eve, 95
listening, 123–24, 139
Long Day's Journey into Night
(O'Neil), 96
love, 156–58, 159
Lunenfeld, Bruno, viii

M
magnetic dimension, 182
Mailer, Norman, 92
Making Sense of Sex (Barash and
Lipton), 95
male menopause: definition of, 2,
31, 32; duration, 37–39;
emotional symptoms, 5, 35;
hormonal symptoms, 35;
importance of recognition,
41–44, 86, 110–11;
interpersonal symptoms, 35;
physical symptoms, 5, 16, 35;
sexual symptoms, 6, 35;
similarities to menopause, 107,
108–9, 138; social symptoms,
35; spiritual symptoms, 35;
statistics, 5, 39
Male Menopause (Diamond),
vii, viii, x, 1
manhood, x, 92–96, 106
ManKind Project, 105, 163
Manson, JoAnn E., 145

marriage, 2, 60, 183
Massachusetts Male Aging
Study, 72
Maximize Your Vitality & Potency
(Wright and Lenard), 144
medication: role in ED, 73
melatonin, 146
memory loss, 5
men: "acting out", 63; behavior
changes in super-adulthood,
182–83; feelings of
vulnerability, 62; need for
support, 29, 54, 63, 92, 104,
161–63, 184; reasons for
insecurity, 93–96; relation to
other men, 188–89; seasons of
life, 80–88; similarities to
women, 115; support sources,
162; trouble reaching out,
116, 117, 128–30
Men's Health Network, 116
men's organizations, 163. *See
also* individual organizations
menopause, female, 116
Menopause: A Positive Approach
(Reitz), 44, 115
mentoring, 104, 106, 175–76,
190–191
middlescence, 89–92
midlife crisis, x: differences
from male menopause, 40
Million Man March, 163

About the Author

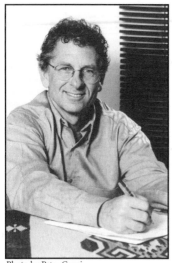

Photo by Peter Carni

Jed Diamond is Director of MenAlive, a health center for men and the women who love them. Since its inception in 1992, Jed has been on the board of advisors of the Men's Health Network, which was established to increase public awareness about the social and economic costs of declining health among men. Diamond has been a licensed psychotherapist for thirty-five years and is an internationally recognized educator and trainer in the area of men's health, gender reconciliation, and addiction prevention and treatment.

He is the author of *Male Menopause,* which has been translated into eleven languages. Diamond also has written three other books, nine booklets, produced ten audio cassette programs, and a video program for the Public Broadcasting System (PBS).

He received his master's degree in social work from the University of California at Berkeley. He is now on the faculty of J.F.K. University, where he offers classes through the Department of Graduate Psychology. He has taught classes at U.C. Berkeley, U.C.L.A., U.C. Santa Barbara, U.C. Santa Cruz, Esalen Institute, the Omega Institute, and other centers of education throughout the country.

He lives with his wife, Carlin, in northern California. They are proud parents of five grown children and seven grandchildren.